...plementing community care

Edited by Nigel A. Malin

Open University Press
Celtic Court
22 Ballmoor
Buckingham
MK18 1XW

and
1900 Frost Road, Suite 101
Bristol, PA 19007, USA

First Published 1994
Reprinted 1994, 1995

A catalogue record of this book is available from the British Library

ISBN 0 335 15738 6 (pb)   0 335 15739 4

Library of Congress Cataloging-in-Publication Data

Implementing community care / edited by Nigel A. Malin.
    p.   cm.
    Includes bibliographical references and index.
    ISBN 0–335–15739–4. — ISBN 0–335–15738–6 (pbk.)
    1. Handicapped—Care—Great Britain.   2. Handicapped–
–Deinstitutionalization—Great Britain.   I. Malin, Nigel.
HV1559.G6I46   1994
362.4′0485—dc20   93–42337
                                                              CIP

Typeset by Graphicraft Typesetters Ltd, Hong Kong
Printed in Great Britain by St Edmundsbury Press Ltd,
Bury St Edmunds, Suffolk

Contents

Preface

This book provides information for those with an interest in community care policy and how it has developed. The individual chapters discuss specific aspects of the Community Care Act 1990 – planning, care management, finance, empowerment, quality – providing relevant background reading. The National Health Service (NHS) Management Executive has in August 1993 set up a Community Care Unit with a remit to monitor the impact of new arrangements on the NHS, to offer support on emerging implementation issues and to run a development programme to generate assistance in taking forward the community care agenda. The intention is to achieve better integration of community care with other strategic policy issues.

It is important that community care succeeds: too many people still remain resident in long-stay hospitals, carers receive limited support, and there are inadequate community residential, day and support services. A much clearer direction from the centre is needed to guide and fund local agencies, to monitor local services and to improve the quality of care. In many ways, government 'market' policy has overtaken principles to supply a genuine humanitarian service. The logic of the new reforms is that individuals should be entitled to a range of services designed within limits to meet their needs. In practice, people with disabilities, mental health problems, etc., will have their needs assessed, a plan defined and maybe little more. Social service departments and health authorities are now forced to operate under very severe restraints and to make maximum use of the independent sector. Their role as planners and adjudicators on community care should in theory encompass the rights of individuals. Yet such rights to services are still not enshrined in practice. Identifying a person's needs has taken on a quality of its own, with the expectation of much stronger user involvement and control in the future.

Acknowledgements

I should like to thank Joan Malherbe and Jacinta Evans of Open University Press, who have given great support throughout, Margaret Bright, Zoe Gibson and Elaine Smith for typing the manuscript, and my colleagues at Sheffield Hallam University for their help and encouragement. I am also grateful to my students, past and present, for the interest they have shown in this area.

I hope this book will be of use to professionals and others in the development of community care services.

Nigel Malin

Notes on contributors

Andy Alaszewski is a Professor of Health Studies and Director of the Institute of Health Studies at the University of Hull. He has been involved in research on the development of policies and services for people with learning disabilities since 1972. His doctoral thesis from the University of Cambridge was published in 1986 by Croom Helm (*Institutional Care and the Mentally Handicapped*). A revised edition of his original North Humberside survey of services for mothers caring for children with learning disabilities was also published in 1986 by Croom Helm (S. Ayer and A. Alaszewski, *Community Care and the Mentally Handicapped*). His Department of Health funded study into the development of an alternative model of care for children with profound learning disabilities was published in 1990 by Routledge (A. Alaszewski and B.M. Ong, *Normalisation in Practice*).

Michael Beazley works for the Social Services Inspectorate of the Department of Health. His career in social services began at age 17, when he joined the Cyrenians as a voluntary residential worker in London. After basic training he went on to work in Lancashire with people who have learning disabilities and later moved to Glasgow, qualifying as a social work teacher and contributing to the West of Scotland Certificate in Social Services Scheme. In 1982, he moved to Bristol where he held a number of management posts with Avon Social Services. He joined the Social Services Inspectorate in 1989 and now works in its Policy and Business Division, with particular responsibilities for community care in the North of England.

John Brown is Lecturer in Social Policy at the University of York. Since 1978 he has been responsible for a continuously funded research programme, involving some 30 grants, into various aspects of staff training in learning disabilities. He is Director of Studies for two postgraduate programmes – the MA in Services for People with Learning Disabilities for middle/senior managers, and the Diploma in Health Services Management for hospital consultants. His publications reflect these research and teaching activities.

David Challis worked as a social worker in mental health services in Lancashire and Salford. He trained as a psychiatric social worker in Manchester and has been educated at the Universities of York, Manchester and Kent. Since 1976 he has worked at the Personal Social Services Research Unit at the University of Kent, where he is currently Reader in Social Work and Social Care and Assistant Director. He is the author of numerous books and articles on care management and has worked on the development and evaluation of services for elderly people for some years. His publications include *Case Management in Community Care* (with B. Davies, Gower, 1986).

Brian Hardy is a Senior Research Fellow in the Community Care Division of the Nuffield Institute of Health, University of Leeds. In recent years, he has collaborated with Gerald Wistow on a series of studies of inter-agency relationships and a number of associated books and articles on joint planning and joint management. He is currently engaged on a long-term study of the mixed economy of social care and, for the second year, an analysis of community care plans commissioned by the Department of Health.

Bob Hudson is a Senior Lecturer in Social Policy at New College Durham and Visiting Fellow in Community Care Studies at the Institute of Health Studies, University of Durham. He has also had a spell as a Visiting Fellow at the King's Fund Institute, London. He lectures on professional courses for those working in health and social services, as well as undertaking a range of consultancy work in community care. He writes regularly in the weekly press and academic quarterlies, and is currently editing a new series of books on Health and Community Care in the 1990s.

Aileen McIntosh is a Research Associate in the Department of Public Health Medicine and a part-time lecturer in the School of Social and Political Sciences at the University of Hull. Between 1989 and 1992, she had an Economic and Social Research Council studentship to undertake a study of the family care of children with learning disabilities under the supervision of Andy Alaszewski. She has recently been involved in research into informal learning among professionals.

Steve McNally is a Lecturer Practitioner with Oxford Brookes University and the Oxfordshire Learning Disability NHS Trust. He has worked in the learning disability field since 1980, including five years as a community nurse. His current role involves teaching students taking the BA (Hons)

Nursing course. He continues to work in partnership with adults who have a learning disability, their families and other workers. Steve acts as an adviser to the Banbury Advocacy Group. His research interests include eliciting service users' views and discovering how people with learning disabilities can be empowered in taking control of their lives.

Nigel Malin has conducted research at the Universities of Sheffield and Strathclyde concerning community care and learning disabilities. Since 1981 he has taught social policy at Sheffield Hallam University where he is Reader in Community Care. In recent years, he has undertaken a number of externally funded research and development projects connected with staff training and the impact of policy on professional practice in community care. He is author of many publications in these areas including editor of *Reassessing Community Care* (Routledge, 1987). He is currently engaged in research on care management for people with learning disabilities.

Jill Manthorpe is Lecturer in Social Work at the University of Hull. She is particularly interested in welfare services for families and individuals and has published in the area of elder abuse, multidisciplinary working, carers' groups and service evaluation. She is currently involved in a variety of community care courses for social workers and community nurses, focusing on adult services and links between policies and practice. Her research focuses mainly on older people, their rights and service developments. Prior to teaching at the University of Hull, she worked in a large voluntary organization and a small urban-aid project.

Jim Monach is Lecturer in Mental Health Studies at the University of Sheffield and Chair of Sheffield MIND. After taking a degree in Sociology, he spent some time as a psychiatric nurse before becoming a psychiatric social worker. After qualifying in social work, he worked in Australia, Sheffield and Derbyshire in both generic and specialist social work posts with local authorities. His particular interests are in mental health issues pursued via teaching, writing, research, MIND and involvement with various community services. Jim is also involved in research and publications in relation to infertility and primary care counselling.

Len Spriggs is an Education Adviser in the Department of Student Guidance at Sheffield Hallam University. He is also Chair of Sheffield Citizen Advocacy (for people with learning difficulties) and Secretary/Deputy Chair of Sheffield MIND. His principal academic interests are in the areas of mental health and learning difficulties, and his current research activities include an evaluation of the Volunteer Training Programme for the Special Olympics, Sheffield 1993 (for Trent Regional Health Authority), and a study of users' experiences of mental health services. His other research interests include mental health promotion and attitudes towards disability.

John Rose is a Clinical Psychologist and Tutor on the South Wales Training Course in Clinical Psychology, based at Whitchurch Hospital, Cardiff. Prior to his move to South Wales, he was active in the implementation of community care legislation in Oxfordshire, attempting to ensure close cooperation between agencies. He has wide-ranging interests in the field of learning disabilities and has published work on topics including sexuality, staff stress, day services and consumer satisfaction.

Gerald Wistow is Professor of Health and Social Care at the Nuffield Institute of Health, Leeds University. He is the co-author of ten books and many other publications about the health and personal social services. He has a special interest in community care planning, wrote the Department of Health Implementation Document in the subject and has led two national surveys of the plans.

Wai-Ling Wun is a Research Associate in the Centre for Research and Information into Mental Disability, University of Birmingham. She is a qualified occupational therapist from Hong Kong. She holds a MSc in Health Administration and Research from the University of Hull and is registered for a PhD in the Department of Psychiatry, University of Birmingham. Her current research interests include the outcome of resettlement of people from long-stay mental handicap hospitals, and service development for children and adults with a learning disability.

Section 1

The policy context

1 Development of community care

Nigel Malin

The history of community care policy could be described as a patchwork of broken promises and moral posturing: government and service agencies asserting the priority of community care and the need to take firm action; evidence from users and carers showing their poor quality of life and difficulties of surviving without support. Central government direction in planning and financing community care has been long awaited. From the late 1980s there has been a turn of events: the Griffiths Report (1988), the White Paper *Caring for People* (Department of Health, 1989a) and the National Health Service and Community Care Act 1990 (the first piece of comprehensive legislation). These have helped to place community care high on a national agenda of health and social policy.

Although much welcomed, it is evidently a cause of displeasure to those committed to improvements in the lives of individuals who would benefit – 'those affected by problems of ageing, mental illness, mental handicap or physical or sensory disability' (*Caring for People*, para. 1.1) – that it is now more than thirty years since the Royal Commission on Mental Illness and Mental Deficiency first recommended the expansion of such services. The intervening years have witnessed one government report following another, structural changes to health and social services, a steady and continuing growth of research and cries from the media on the depth of the problem. So why hasn't enough been done? Is community care an unpopular political cause? Inspired guesswork would suggest that it is: all political parties support it but have been unwilling to commit necessary resources to implement it. In a political climate where all welfare expenditure is being evaluated, weak, vulnerable and disadvantaged members of society appear to suffer relatively higher losses. The government's drive during the last decade to divest public sector agencies of their ability to plan for the needs of local populations has set one group against another – professional groups, managers, users, carers and campaigners.

It is not clear the extent to which resources to support people should be wholly or partly financial or in kind. Neither government nor statutory local providers are committed, for example, to granting cash payments to individuals to set up home in the community or to buy their own day-care support. In most cases, limited services are available from which an individual may choose (if in fact any choice exists). The new reforms still pose problems on this front:

> Although the calculation [of grant] transfers existing expenditure and even allows for some growth, it does not appear to include provision for the extension of care to those people whose needs are currently neglected, unless efficiency savings release resources for this purpose. This runs the risk of perpetuating some of the inadequacies of the existing arrangements and threatens the success of the new.
>
> (House of Commons Health Committee, 1993a: para. 57)

Martin Knapp claims that cost considerations have always been important in the planning of social care services and that 'their importance can hardly have been more pressing or more widely acknowledged than in recent years' (Knapp, 1993). He argues that the cost of community care remains one of the most oversimplified and under-studied concepts in the lexicon of social care planning: the need to distinguish costs from prices, both as constructs and in their usage, and that an opportunity costing approach would highlight the deviations. The systems and incentives promoted by the National Health Service and Community Care Act require a different approach to service planning and delivery. Ideally, as the Act, its antecedent White Papers and its later guidance and implementation documents make plain, health and social care decision-making will be bottom-up, needs-led and multiple-agency, with innovations encouraged by financial and other incentives, and system implications couched in terms of social and not merely public expenditures. 'The nature and intensity of the cost information requirements of the 1990s will be rather different from those of previous decades' (Knapp et al., 1993).

The purpose of this first chapter is two-fold: to trace the recent phase of policy development to the formal introduction of the Community Care Act 1993 and to consider some of the implications for services and for staff who have responsibility for implementing the reforms.

Has central government direction been mean or modest?

Since Sir Roy Griffiths first published his report (*Community Care: Agenda for Action*, 1988) supporting a mixed economy and the development and regulation of community care, cynics have feared the worst. For many, there was a sense of fulfilment – a plan of action with a focus on organizational structures combined with user aspirations. For others, more realistically grounded perhaps, this heralded the advent of possibilities – where ideas were shaped but where the final outcome for those who needed community care most would be restricted by a whole range of factors (Glendinning, 1988; Lunn 1988; Croft and Beresford, 1989; Hepplewhite, 1989; Phillips, 1989; Ward 1990).

The Griffiths Report (1988)

The week this was issued, the claim was that 'Local Authorities ha(d) emerged from Sir Roy Griffiths' review of community care with a new lease of life. Though that might ensure his report is already in ministers' dustbins, he is adamant that social services departments should take the initiative in providing welfare in the community' (Davies, 1988). Soon after, David Hunter and Ken Judge in a briefing paper suggested that the Griffiths proposals posed a number of major challenges and opportunities and that it was not clear whether central or local government was equipped to meet them. Doubts they stated emerged over:

- central government's willingness to provide policy leadership and ability to undertake the major executive task of monitoring and approving detailed local plans
- central government's willingness to delegate new responsibilities to local authorities
- social services departments' ability to assume the new roles proposed by Griffiths
- social services departments' commitment to community care for the priority groups

(Hunter and Judge, 1988)

Griffiths did not address levels of resources for community care but acknowledged that having ambitious policy goals without the means to implement them was the worst of all possible worlds. Modernizing the management of community care was seen as more important than changing the organization: 'If community care means anything it is that responsibility is placed as near to the individual and his carers as possible' (Griffiths, 1988: para. 30).

At the centre of the framework, Griffiths proposed a minister for community care who would link national policy more clearly to resources and timetables. The minister would be responsible for monitoring local and national policies, ensuring that they are consistent and up to standard. But social services authorities should be left responsible for deciding the content of the plans themselves. The report stressed the mixed economy of care, arguing that it was not necessary for social services authorities to provide all services themselves, simply to ensure that they are provided.

They should act 'as the designers, organisers and purchasers of non-healthcare services and not primarily as direct service providers, making the maximum possible use of voluntary and private sector bodies to widen consumer choice, stimulate innovation, and encourage efficiency' (Griffiths, 1988: para. 1.3.4).

Griffiths argued that their role would become one of case management, assessing the gap between resources and individual needs, targeting funds to devise cost-effective care packages and regularly reviewing priorities. The role of 'health' care (as opposed to social care) was never defined satisfactorily but complementarity of purpose was nevertheless desired. Radical changes in the workforce were needed, involving significant changes in role for a number of professional and occupational groups. There was a further argument taken up from a previous Audit Commission report (1986) recommending the creation of a new occupation of 'community carers' to undertake 'the front-line personal and social support of dependent people' (Griffiths, 1988: para. 8.4). This provided a case for developing new skills among existing staff to enable them to tackle the new tasks proposed, to develop completely new roles and to replace those that no longer appeared to be necessary.

The 1989 White Paper

The 1989 White Paper, *Caring for People* (Department of Health, 1989a) constituted the formal government response to Griffiths, and taken together with *Working for Patients* (Department of Health, 1989b), set out how the government envisaged health and social services would develop over the 1990s and beyond. There were six key objectives:

- to promote the development of domiciliary, day and respite services to enable people to live in their own homes wherever feasible and sensible;
- to ensure service providers make practical support for carers a high priority;
- to make the proper assessment of need and good case management the cornerstone of high-quality care;
- to promote the development of a flourishing independent sector alongside quality public services;
- to clarify the responsibilities of agencies and so make it easier to hold them to account for their performance;
- to secure better value for taxpayers' money by introducing a funding structure for social care.

The prime focus was upon the reform of the organization and funding of social care as NHS responsibilities seemed to remain unaltered but of fundamental importance strategically, for example in compiling care packages. The White Paper stated how the primary health care team had a vital role to play, as general practitioners (GPs) would remain the first port of call for people in the community and '[would] contrive to meet most of their basic healthcare needs'. Social services authorities would need to strengthen their existing management arrangements, particularly with regard to planning, accountability, financial control, purchasing and quality control systems and would be expected to 'make maximum possible use of independent providers of residential and nursing home care when arranging placements'. The view of the government was that the intro-duction of competitive tendering to residential and nursing homes would enhance the ability of social services authorities to obtain best value for public money.

Some of the major critiques of the White Paper have examined the establishment of planning, assessment and care management (Beardshaw and Towell, 1990; Langan, 1990; Cheetham, 1991). While the document argued for 'simplicity as the key', establishing objectives, organization and support mechanisms has been seen as complex and challenging. Para-graph 5.10 specifies that 'SSDs [would be] expected to set out the needs of the population they service'. Elsewhere in the White Paper there is the direction that carers' needs must be explicitly assessed. Implicit is the recognition of carers not simply as a means to an end – more community care – but ends in themselves with their own needs and rights to welfare. For the past decade, as commentators have recognized (Cheetham, 1991; Wistow, 1993), needs assessment has not been high on the agenda in both research and policy. In its assault on dependency, the government has discouraged such investigations and thereby the ensuing call for more resources.

Caring for People stated that social services authorities would be respons-ible for designing care packages to meet individual needs, in consultation with clients and other professionals, and 'within available resources'. It gives the government's view that:

> Where an individual's needs are complex or significant levels of re-sources are involved . . . [there is] considerable merit in nominating a casemanager [later termed caremanager] . . . to take responsibility for ensuring that individuals' needs are regularly reviewed, resources are managed effectively and that each service user has a single point of contact . . . Case management provides an effective method of targeting resources and planning services to meet specific needs of individual clients.
>
> (Department of Health, 1989a: paras 3.3.2 and 3.3.3)

The White Paper asserted that care managers would often be employed by the social services authority but that this 'need not always be so' (para. 3.3.2). It listed elements of effective care management as including:

- identification of people in need, including systems for referral
- assessment of care needs
- planning and securing the delivery of care
- monitoring the quality of care provided
- review of client needs

(Department of Health, 1989a: para. 3.3.4)

While it was not essential that the same manager undertake all these tasks for a particular client, a clearly identified individual should be designated for each function. The White Paper suggested a range of backgrounds for care managers, with social workers, home care managers or community nurses as possibly the most suitable (para. 3.3.4). It gave the government's view that there was an advantage in linking care management with delegated responsibility for budgetary management as 'an important way of enabling those closest to the identification of client needs to make the best possible use of the resources available' (para. 3.3.6). It then would be left to in-dividual authorities to indicate how they proposed to employ care man-agement techniques and develop clear budgetary systems (Beardshaw and Towell, 1990).

The Community Care Act (as part of the National Health Service and Community Care Act 1990)

When the Community Care Act went through Parliament, there was con-siderable – but unsuccessful – pressure to provide ringfenced funding. The reforms were delayed because of government fears that they would add thirty pence per week to poll tax bills (Massie, 1992). Essentially, the Act replicates the framework of the White Paper but is short on its com-mitments, mainly confined to user rights to assessment and a care plan. It makes no provision, for example, for authorized representation of dis-abled people who are unable to put their own case, nor does it require local authorities to be accountable by giving reasons for not providing a service.

    The Act was marooned for two years (as the expected date for full implementation was April 1991). During this period, the Institute for Health Service Management (1992), as one of several professional bodies, criti-cized the Department of Health for not funding or planning the changes adequately. It claimed confusion between health and local authorities, as they would not be fully ready to implement the new system by April 1993. Managers accused the Department of Health of lack of clarity about what it would expect and complained of uncertain guidance over joint planning. The Act was designed to blur boundaries, inspire confidence and clarify the various tasks required by the new relationship between health and local authority employees, but increasing evidence showed how this objective was not being realized. A report by the Audit Commission (1992), *Homeward Bound: A New Course for Community Health*, drew attention to difficulties that could arise if health and social care were not clearly defined. It argued for district health authorities to provide extra nursing support for people leaving residential care (although this was now seen as a local authority issue) and that joint consultative committees consistently failed to produce policies that met the needs of people with disabilities, elderly people and those discharged from hospital.

There have been concerns over the meaning and force of the legislation: it has been left for the individual agencies to interpret. An intended objective is 'to solve many of the problems of the past by establishing a new relationship between health and local authorities and between service providers and recipients' (John, 1993). The legislation requires local authorities to make assessments and to draw up individual care plans for patients being discharged from hospitals and for other vulnerable people who are able to live in the community.

The Community Care Act does not replace existing duties and powers but creates new duties for social services departments. It links an evaluation of an individual's needs for a service to an authority's decision whether to provide it or not. Section 47 is general and brief but summarizes potential service applicants' new rights as: a right to an assessment and, where an assessment is carried out, a right to a 'decision' on providing community care services. The assessment right arises 'where it appears to a local authority that any person for whom they may provide . . . community care services may be in need of any such services' (section 47(1)). The right to a decision arises because the authority 'having regard to the results of [the] assessment, shall then decide whether [the person's] needs call for the provision by them of any . . . services' (section 47(1) (b)). Where it appears that the person is a 'disabled person' and possibly entitled to services under section 2 of the Chronically Sick and Disabled Persons Act 1970, the authority has also to decide whether to provide such services (section 47(2)). The absence of prescriptive guidance leaves worries about entitlement, at best ambiguous, at worst confusingly unresolved (Bynoe, 1993). It is not clear whether there is any duty to provide a service once an assessment has shown the need for it, as local authorities may still claim that resources remain insufficient to provide for all assessed needs.

In preparation for implementation of the Act, local community care plans needed to be submitted by April 1992 relating to services in 1993–94 onwards. Howard Glennerster, criticizing Department of Health draft guidance on planning as being 'vacuous and unhelpful', identified broad principles that should underlie needs-based planning: think beyond your own department, think in client group terms, think about multiple futures, needs and realistic resource constraints and consult the consumers:

> Need categories and the expected numbers in each must be sufficiently detailed for an interdisciplinary group that includes carers and advocates or users, to be able to discuss representative cases realistically and arrive at a set of agreed packages of care. *These can then be costed and multiplied up to give a total expenditure implied if each subgroup were to get the most effective set of caring packages the group agree on.*
>
> (Glennerster, 1991; my emphasis)

The Act demands that local services should set up a basis for identifying and costing the needs of individuals requiring community care; this would be followed by supply-side developments and dialogue with users on how much each person can afford.

Health Secretary William Waldegrave, speaking at a conference in Eastbourne in September 1991, pledged that resourcing for community care would be presented 'in a way that shows how much extra goes to local authorities by transfer from social security . . . we shall make sure that local government and any others with an interest can see exactly how the sums are done'. A Whitehall web of committees (later known as the Algebra Group) were engaged to investigate global sums of money that the Department of Social Security (DSS) would have to pay out in income support and attendance allowance if the (then) present system of payments for residential care was to be sustained. The Association of Metropolitan Authorities (AMA) estimated a £300 million shortfall between income support levels and the amount elderly people actually have to pay for places in residential homes. The (then) DSS Minister Ann Widdicombe expressed the government's dilemma perfectly when rejecting the suggestion (BBC *PM Programme*, 14 November 1991). If the government simply made up the shortfall, it would have no way of controlling private homes costs. The argument was that DSS officers did not have a competency to judge what those costs should be, but from April 1993 local authorities would, in theory, have that competency.

Other indicators stressed that elderly people's savings were being unacceptably swallowed up by the high costs of private residential care and falling public services and that only 10 per cent of people over seventy were able to purchase their own care, requiring a disposable income of at least double the income support level (Counsel and Care, 1991; Oldham, 1991). Under present legislative conditions, if a person gives away their home, for example, to a relative six months or more before making a request to the local authority for residential care, then neither the person concerned nor family member becomes liable to contribute to residential home fees.

Table 1 Community care special transitional grant

Year	Amount (£ million)	Comment
1993–94	£565	DSS transfer plus £140 m additional funding plus £26.8 m 'ILF' money
1994–95	£716	Increase in transfer plus £64.1 m 'ILF'
1995–96	£618	Increase in transfer plus £99.9 m 'ILF'
1996–97	Phase out	

Note: Apart from the ILF element, each year's grant goes into the subsequent year's SSA baseline.
Source: Department of Health (1993).

Financing the reforms

The 1989 White Paper made clear that finance for local authorities' new community care responsibilities would be channelled through the revenue support grant and distributed between authorities in the normal way on the basis of their standard spending assessment (SSA). However, the government concluded that there was a case for modifying these principles in the early years of the policy and decided to introduce a ringfenced special transitional grant (STG). The original grant was announced on 2 October 1992; it was later announced that a further amount would be included to recognize new burdens on local authorities as a result of changes to the Independent Living Fund (ILF). Table 1 summarizes these amounts.

The majority of funding consisted of monies transferred from the social security budget already supporting those using residential services; relatively small amounts were to support changes in social services' infrastructure or for developing new projects. Key features of the STG were that the grant would be for a four-year transitional period, that it would be ringfenced for use on community care services and directly related activities, be outside capping calculations and have a special transitional distribution formula. In the first year, the grant would include monies transferred from the DSS to local authorities in respect of their new responsibilities (£399 million). The second and third years would include the increase in the social security transfer and the whole of the ILF amount, phasing out in the fourth year. In each case, the previous year's grant would be added to the social service's SSA baseline, meaning that over time an increasing proportion of funding for community care would be through the normal standard spending assessment.

The DSS transfer element of the STG was to be distributed among local authorities, half according to the existing pattern of DSS spending on income support in independent residential and nursing home provision, and half according to revised SSA calculations which are capitation-based and intended to reflect need in the whole population for which the local authority is responsible. The £140 million portion of the STG was to be distributed according to this SSA formula. Therefore, 37 per cent of the total STG in 1993–94 would be distributed according to current DSS spending and 63 per cent according to SSA.

A precondition of receiving payment was for local authorities to provide evidence of joint agreements with health authorities by 31 December 1992 on: (1) strategies governing health and local authorities' responsibilities for placing people in nursing homes, and the numbers likely to be involved during 1993–94; and (2) agreement as to how hospital discharge arrangements will be integrated with assessment arrangements. All 108 local authorities in England met this deadline, as the Parliamentary Under Secretary phrased it, 'for delivering proof of their partnership agreements with health authorities' (Department of Health Press Release H93/476).

The government originally proposed an additional condition that at least 75 per cent of each local authority's total grant was to be spent in the independent sector. Seventy-five per cent of the STG in fact amounted to £404 million, which was slightly more than the £399 million that constituted the DSS transfer element of the grant. In effect this meant that, according to the Local Authority Associations' (LAA) own calculations, some local authorities' share of the DSS transfer would amount to less than 75 per cent of their total grant, meaning that a proportion of their share of the £140 million would be required to meet this shortfall. After discussions with the LAAs and others, the requirement was changed to 85 per cent of the DSS transfer element. This works out as 64 per cent of the total grant, somewhat less than the original 75 per cent figure. Local authorities had to demonstrate that they would spend 85 per cent over and above their baseline personal social services' (PSS) expenditure on the 'independent sector', which was defined for these purposes as 'meaning not under local authority ownership, management or control' (House of Commons Health Committee, 1993a).

If community care policy was to succeed in its aim of providing more appropriate care for individuals in more homely settings, local authorities would need to commission an increasing proportion of community-based care packages. The NHS would have an enhanced contribution to make by ensuring that the relevant health components of these packages, such as district nursing, community psychiatric nursing, health visiting, physiotherapy and chiropody, were provided. Among the uses of an additional £800 million announced by the Department of Health for 1993–94 was that of providing extra support for community health services so that the NHS could play its part in implementing the changes. From April 1993, general practice fundholders would be able to purchase community health services and would therefore have a significant part to play in the planning and commissioning of appropriate community care services. Their budgets for purchasing these services would be based on an assessment of how much the relevant district health authority spent on their patients for community health services in 1992–93.

The House of Commons Health Committee Third Report (*Community Care: Funding from April 1993*) assessed the extent to which the government's claim that the criteria for the funding settlement would be 'transparent, adequate and fair' (para. 24) had been met.

Transparency The Report claimed that the Department of Health 'ha[d] not explained the relative weighting it ha[d] given to the factors used in calculating the rate of increase of new residents' (para. 41) and that in relation to the additional £140 million for start-up costs the sum had been chosen at random (para. 43). The £140 million would be a recurrent sum subsumed in baseline SSAs but in practice demand for some of the elements for which it was intended, such as assessment, reassessment and respite care, would increase in subsequent years. The LAAs estimated that to cover the shortfall between Income Support and homes' fees alone, £66 million would be required, thus depleting by nearly half the £140 million allocated by the Department of Health for many more functions besides meeting this shortfall. The government's response, published in May 1993, stated:

The £40 million additional funding is the Government's judgement of what local authorities will need above the transfer from the Department of Social Security to carry out their new community care responsibilities. The Committee may wish to know that the factors taken into account included costs arising from development of purchasing and contracting, costs of care, development of financial systems, assessment and caremanagement, information technology, the effect of the alignment of charges, home care and support to carers and top up payments to those with preserved rights under pension age. *It is not the Government's practice to give a detailed breakdown of the components of allocations to local authorities for personal social services, in this case particularly in view of the very great differences that exist among local authorities, and their differing needs and priorities with regard to the items listed.*

(Departments of Health and Social Security, 1993:
para. 4, p. 6; my emphasis)

Adequacy Most of the written evidence received during the Health Committee's inquiry referred to the shortfall between Income Support and homes' fees (House of Commons Health Committee, 1993a: para. 66). The problems identified included concerns about the future for residents and their relatives who could no longer afford to 'top-up' and the future of charities facing financial hardships. Local authorities made some use of their power to 'top-up' for residents under pension age, although it was illegal for them to do the same for older residents. Some district health authorities also topped up people with learning disabilities in independent sector homes who have been discharged from long-stay hospitals. A *Guardian* survey in 1993 showed that the number of NHS beds for elderly people with long-term illnesses had been cut by nearly 40 per cent since 1988, forcing people into means-tested private nursing homes (in total more than 10 000 beds had been closed). The means-testing regulations for private nursing home fees have meant that people with assets of more than £8000, including their homes, receive no financial help. As a result, nursing care has been financed by house sales.

Evidence has shown that in 1993–94 the gap between the Department of Health's and the LAAs' calculations of total funding requirements was £289 million, comprising £90 million for the DSS transfer, £145 million for the difference between Income Support and homes' charges and £54 million for support and other service costs. These figures were later revised to take account of inflation forecasts, benefit level uprating (1993–94) and the announcement that £26 million would be grantable to local authorities to replace the ILF. This showed a reduced overall gap of £138 million: £62 million arising from the DSS transfer, £66 million for the shortfall between benefits and charges and £10 million for support and other costs.

On the question of unmet need, the committee recommended that 'clear guidance be issued urgently to local authorities . . . and, if necessary, legislation introduced to make sure that there are no inhibitions on the ability of social services' departments and health authorities to make a full assessment of unmet needs. It will be difficult to judge in the future whether resources are adequate unless we have a clear indication of the level of need, both met and unmet' (para. 64). The government response was equivocal, claiming that it was up to authorities to set out clearly their priorities and eligibility criteria for services and to collect the evidence they needed for planning purposes (para. 7, p. 7).

Fairness   The House of Commons Health Committee (1993a) asserted that the way in which resources for community care should be allocated would hinge on the twin effects of the distribution formula and the requirement that at least 85 per cent of each local authority's transfer must be spent on the independent sector. The distribution of the STG to individual local authorities was determined by 'the 50 : 50 formula for the DSS transfer, half according to current social security expenditure and half according to SSA' (para. 111), and viewed as a compromise (in the absence of more robust data), based both on current patterns of provision and need as calculated by SSAs. The Association of Metropolitan Authorities (AMA) criticized the formula, as authorities with low levels of independent provision would be penalized were resources to be distributed according to current provision, not need. The formula did not include migration data (information on claimants' original residence) and would discriminate against authorities where the independent sector had been underdeveloped due to higher costs rather than lower levels of need.

In its evidence, the National Institute of Social Work (NISW) claimed that '[this would] of course reinforce existing inequalities in favour of wealthier areas and at the expense of poorer ones. Poorer areas need to build up local services (whether residential or domiciliary) if people in those areas were to be able to continue to live there, rather than being shipped out to residential care elsewhere' (Evidence to House of Commons Health Committee, 1993a: Vol. II, para. 95). The committee suggested maintaining the consequences of the 50 : 50 distribution formula to clarify its impact – the government rejected this proposal stating that it was not feasible to undertake this 'in isolation from other factors' (Departments of Health and Social Security, 1993: para. 18).

Does a service infrastructure exist to undertake community care successfully?

In September 1992, a community care task force was set up by the NHS management executive focusing upon a number of local authorities (*c.* 20) where the Department of Health appeared to have cause for concern about their lack of preparation for the reforms. It would usually arrange for a team of five to eight of its members with a mix of skills and background to spend one day fact-finding and give feedback. The approach was described as holistic – looking at the social services department's work with the health authority, the Family Health Service Authority (FHSA) and the private and voluntary sectors (King, 1993). The most common blockages found were a lack of an identified social services person in overall charge (often SSDs had several people leading different bits of implementation or more than one person thought they were in charge), implementation had started too late and relationships with the independent and voluntary sector were very weak. An important part of the task force's job was to collect and disseminate examples of good practice.

The consequences of reforms for staff are considerable as changes to existing functions have been identified (Common and Flynn, 1992; George, 1993; Malin, 1993b; Teasdale, 1993). Care management skills, for example, have caused problems: some qualified and experienced professionals fear core assessment by a broader range of workers undermines their skills and devalues their training. Specific training in care management roles could resolve these concerns, but some fieldwork staff have felt training had been too little, too late (Hoyes and Means, 1993). The White Paper (Department of Health, 1989a) took the view that 'social services authorities [would] need to give careful consideration to the training and development of management, planning and front-line staff to fulfil [their] roles . . . particularly in developing common understanding and joint working arrangements for care management and assessment (para. 11.45). For the professional worker, the introduction and development of the contract culture has had three consequences: employer-led training, new patterns of demarcation and the introduction of alternative qualifications. 'By the end of [the 1980s] the concept of joint training had become an essential part of the government's strategy to promote integrated services in community care' (Brown, 1992).

Workforce planning and staff training

Training may be widely recognized as a foundation stone for the successful implementation of community care, although developments at local level have been mixed and partial. Only one month before the 1993 implementation date, many social services departments and social work departments (SWDs) in Scotland were still organizing last minute courses on the necessary new skills. Community care training was viewed as much about instilling confidence, allaying anxieties and reinforcing skills as it was about providing specific courses on care management, needs-led assessment and the like (Mitchell, 1993). The Department of Health/Price Waterhouse report on practice guidance stressed that social services' staff required an understanding of how to operate in practice within the mixed economy and published a set of training guidelines for the purchase of services (DoH/SSI/LBTC, 1992). This followed work commissioned by the Central Council for Education and Training in Social Work (CCETSW, 1989, 1992) and the Department of Health Social Services Inspectorate (DoH/SSI, 1990, 1991a) highlighting directions on training need as a consequence of the new legislation. Such concerns are not limited to the domain of SSDs. MacKenzie (1993) has pointed out how community nurses are in a similar dilemma given GP rights to curtail services that district nurses and health visitors can offer, coupled with the drive to identify explicit skills seen as purchasable within a market culture (NHSME, 1992; District Nursing Association, 1993).

Studies singling out training needs for informal carers have shown a lack of commitment for working partnerships on behalf of statutory agencies, illustrating that training when it occurs depends on one-to-one social worker–client contact (Nolan and Grant, 1989: Atkinson and McHaffie, 1992). In 1991, CCETSW (Northern Region) commissioned the York Link Consortium to develop a series of regional conferences to elaborate training needs emerging from the community care legislation with respect to services for people with learning disabilities. The findings were published in a report suggesting that 'experimentation is required to develop training, particularly at post-qualifying level to test out how ideas associated with the new culture (caremanagement, working with the independent sector) would be implemented in practice' (Malin, 1993a). During this period, the Social Services Inspectorate and CCETSW set up a Training Strategy Group to look at joint training at six sites throughout England (DoH/SSI, 1990). They later argued that the purchaser–provider distinction was now more important than the role of professional bodies (DoH/SSI, 1991a).

In 1991, the SSI (Yorkshire and Humberside Region) commissioned a study involving collaboration with two SSDs (North Yorkshire and Bradford) to provide data for training plans and to support the evolution of workforce planning required as a result of changes being introduced by the Community Care Act 1990 (Malin, 1993c). One declared objective was 'to develop methodology for translating strategic plans into estimates for workforce recruitment and training requirements'. Bradford SSD has been in the process of undertaking a training needs analysis (TNA) to identify: key changes in services whose implementation would depend on the retraining of the workforce; decisions about training priorities and the resources committed to these priorities; and management of training and levels of training in relation to particular sections of the workforce including requirements from independent organizations. This is against a not untypical background where professional qualifications are limited, particularly in residential, day and domiciliary care, and where there is an absence of new initiatives to address ideas raised by the legislation. The training plan set as a goal:

> ... a need to develop managers to lead the organisation through changes especially on caremanagement and assessment; furthering systems needed for delivering NVQs; ensuring that all staff are recognised/accredited for training; [and] increasing the proportion of joint training with voluntary, private and health services.
>
> (Bradford Social Services Training Plan, 1992)

The North Yorkshire training plan stated a need to make more use of external training providers and provide a workforce which is more responsive and less prescriptive. Data on the workforce indicated a high incidence of managers in residential and day services with social work, nursing or teaching qualifications (relatively low in homes for older people), and a much lower incidence of similar qualifications among care staff. A criticism was the lack of strategic input addressing community care training whether for carers or social workers.

The evaluation based on analysing training needs of care staff, managers of residential, day and home care units, and social workers fulfilling the care management role, illustrated opportunities for skill transfer in areas of assessment, care planning and working with the independent sector (that is, various members of the workforce had significant levels of relevant skill and experience which could be topped-up to promote a genuine needs-led approach). From interviews with care managers, distinct themes emerged:

1. *The lack of involvement of users in assessment.* Current practice precluded users from involvement in multidisciplinary assessments, as there was a tension between professional assessment of need and demands users made on services. Skills were often limited to assessing need for a specific type of service, such as domiciliary help, as looking at need holistically was a relatively alien concept (less so in the case of the social workers interviewed):

   > We need skills to allow people to express their needs – we go in with a knowledge of what's on offer and make people fit into what you've got. This means allowing people to open up and say what they actually feel they need. Also give them enough information to be able to make a realistic request.
   >
   > (Home care manager)

   They stated how difficult it had been involving users in designing assessment schedules; as a result, this process had lacked user representation. They expressed a need to develop skills on how to empower users in all stages of the assessment process, so that users could contribute towards the outcome of care plans.

2. *The inadequacy of data on user needs.* Care managers mentioned the need for a user database for monitoring service input and outcomes expressed through changes in individual lifestyles.

   > There is a lot of information around but it's not available in any systematic way – it's not retrievable. We react to a demand for services but it's done on the basis of expediency. We don't yet know who needs what and how our resources could be used more effectively.
   >
   > (Social work manager)

   This raises the suggestion that skills are needed to process information and ensure that needs are explicitly revealed in service contracts. In the absence of holistic assessment, referrals were based on limited prescription of information to which providers responded incrementally, such as when a home care manager receives referral for a specific service but having then made her own assessment, suggests a service which may contrast with the original request. This had been a function of working to resources, assigned to separate services, but respondents believed that for the process to work effectively in the interests of users, information should be coordinated, requiring training in prioritizing services and managing the range of inputs embodied within each individual contract.

3. *The need for collaboration among professionals in designing care packages.* Care managers stated that they did not (yet) design care packages and had no formal responsibility for making demands on other services; instead, their role was restricted to collating assessment data to support a method that would be user-friendly. They expressed a need for shared training as a prerequisite to inter-agency agreements, which would include building on shared values, determining eligibility for service and resource allocation.

> Some people are very skilled in some areas and not in others and the differences between staff have to be acknowledged. Current thinking in training seems to be that we can all end up doing all of the jobs, if you like, we are all interchangeable, and I don't think that we are. Different perceptions are needed.
>
> (Social worker)

4. *The need for budgeting skills and information on costings.* There was a general need to be more aware of the cost of services to individual users: departmental costing of in-house services had not been completed, hence it was not possible to cost individual services and not clear how budgets were being devolved. The difficulty is in providing a balance within a restricted budget so that resources are seen to be fairly and evenly distributed, while at the same time making sure that people with special needs, such as those with multiple handicaps, are being addressed. This will mean guidance on priority setting in the context of drawing upon the ability of users to contribute financially and in kind towards the overall cost of their care:

> Well it may be again a function of working to resources – if you talk to a particular lady who is very fastidious about her housework for example, she may actually need four hours a week cleaning. So I would say she doesn't need it, all she needs is [say] two hours and that is based around resources we have available and also my professional judgement. The difference would result in having to find resources from other sources. This would mean the lady taking the initiative and to assist that we would need to ensure that she is aware of all available options.
>
> (Home care manager)

Working to budget was raised as more of a problem for social workers (acting as care managers) than for home care managers who are described as 'having to do it all day every day':

> I think a lot of people who work on the budget-type basis can get
> a bit divorced from the needs of the individual . . . some of them
> will need to develop more understanding of the proactive busi-
> ness of being led by the service user.
>
> (Social worker)

5. *The lack of established criteria ensuring quality standards.* Data presented
under this heading related to describing how services are given or not
given to users despite the absence of any formal means for identifying
need. For example, with day care a range of inputs were provided but
there was no preliminary assessment:

> I want day care for this person to be doing x, y and z requiring
> the service to re-think and restructure itself and actually provide
> a service – I mean they work very hard but they were sort of in
> tramlines with fixed patterns of responding.
>
> (Social worker)

By changing the function of day centres from all-purpose centres to
concentrating on developing professional expertise tailored to individual needs would, it was suggested, be more attractive to the majority
of users. The issue of how to establish standards in care packages was
raised by all interviewees as there were no fixed criteria: 'We agree
monitoring arrangements but it may be necessary to develop a more
structured monitoring procedure'.

Staff had exercised their own judgement as the department had not
yet set out standards on quality practice. This had discouraged them
from raising issues affecting policy decisions and channelling views on
how quality criteria could be included within contracts, which was further affected by poor collaboration with external agencies:

> We can guarantee the input from our own department and from
> what we are buying in from elsewhere; we cannot guarantee the
> health input at all; there's no way of doing that and I don't know
> how we are going to get round that.
>
> (Social worker)

The interviews identified difficulties in undertaking care management
and the existence of training needs in the above areas. Interdisciplinary
training would seem necessary for understanding different roles and for
establishing a common language and terminology – a vital ingredient of
almost all community care plans published in April 1993. Until internal
SSD/Health Authority changes are decided, then the role of care manager remains ambivalent. Within the care management literature, there is
a debate about the style of care management, which may be characterized

as being between 'administrative' and 'clinical' approaches. David Challis (1993) writes:

> Some agencies looking at the core tasks of caremanagement appear to see them rather more as administrative activities than requiring staff with human relations skills. However, the [PSSRU] studies indicate that caremanagement has been successful in performing the core tasks through combining practical care with the use of human relations skills, including counselling and support, not only to carers and users but also to direct care staff. Conversely an 'administrative' approach would be more likely to fragment such activities as resources to be purchased separately where necessary.

Lesley Bell (1993) endorses the need for new skills:

> Care service managers in all sectors need new skills: business planning; financial management; developing tenders to meet specifications; contract negotiation; contract compliance; and marketing and market research. Without these, their agencies or units will not survive in the brave new competitive world of caremanagement, commissioning and contracting, and the separation of purchasing and providing care services.

Staff need to know what constitutes a quality service, what standards are expected and have the competence to achieve them. Yet training and development for service providers has virtually been ignored. The National Vocational Qualification (NVQ) integrated awards may be the way forward for staff, by being based on a national standard of competence required in the workplace (Todd, 1993), and the care management qualification proposed by the Local Government Management Board may be the way forward for service managers. But these will not become readily available and accessible until late 1993 and into 1994. It will take time before any significant impact is made on the quality of the services provided.

To date, most training plans seem geared to immediate needs. As neither CCETSW nor the Department of Health has yet issued clear guidelines on long-term national training structures, there is an expectation of a rather amorphous training continuum from NVQs through qualifying training to post-qualification level. It is not yet clear as to whether social work will be the core component, whether it will be a combination of NVQ social care skills with appropriate management training, or whether an entirely new programme of in-house training will form the basis for most staff.

The marathon of change taking place within services requires new skills to be developed. The SSI has been a major player in issuing guidance on skills for social work and social care staff (DoH/SSI, 1990) and in putting forward a 'joint approach' (DoH/SSI, 1991b). The latter argues for local agencies to formulate a joint service strategy and make training and development an integral part of that strategy, involving the innovative practical support of carers, integrating equal opportunities and anti-discriminatory practices, and developing assessment and care management systems which address consumer needs. Important points for training include involving relevant stakeholders early on in the process, making efforts to engage users and carers, GPs, housing agencies and voluntary not-for-profit and private sector bodies, and ensuring strong and continuing links between strategic management, service providers and trainers so that training becomes owned by managers and by the organization and related directly to service objectives. Guidance from the above places emphasis on 'learning by doing' – setting up pilot projects now, especially in assessment and care management. The intention would be to bring about realistic objectives based on a joint system helping participants to learn about each others' tasks, roles and skills and how they can collaborate in a shared model of care. Both CCETSW and the English National Board for Nursing, Midwifery and Health Visiting (ENB) have been active in supporting shared training throughout the country (Thompson and Mathias, 1992), in the evolution of different models of shared training and in providing funding support.

Workforce planning is a significant aspect of community care, which requires provider agencies to examine staffing (skills, training, expertise) and to match needs with available resources (Edmondston, 1988; Gourlay, 1991). Whichever way people work it is important to look at who does what best. Across the professions, some skills relate to specific anatomical areas. For example, speech therapists generally concentrate on the face and neck areas and chiropodists the feet, while physiotherapists and occupational therapists embrace the whole body. Many professional groups tackle the psychosocial aspects of care. National vocational qualifications will become available for all care staff regardless of whether they are employed by health, voluntary, private or social services. Currently, two types of NVQ are available to the care sector: health care support worker competences and residential, domiciliary and day-care competences. It is important that paid carers cease to see their job as minding, but take on a more active role based on goal planning and support identifying options for work, leisure and educational opportunity. The resource-question simply helps to focus the mind but needs to become the responsibility of all care-givers, not just those who wear a management hat.

Local provider networks

Sir Roy Griffiths, writing in 1992, presented the following dilemma:

> Is the market geared to provide many of the services required? The essence of any market is not simply to provide competition so that

a higher quality and more efficient service emerges, but also to extend the range of choice by innovation and to provide the sheer dynamic to rush in to meet perceived requirements. It is early days, but there is a vast and growing market not only for provision to the statutory authorities and their clients, but directly to the growing body of more affluent people in the community. We have to expect that the private sector can see and meet the opportunities.

This is also the government's view, but in reality there is a fixed limit for providing opportunities through the independent sector. This is not helped by the divisions that remain between health and social care funding (Collins, 1992). Nearly 25 000 people with learning disabilities remain in long-stay hospitals in England. The fact that this number continues to decline is, to a significant extent, due to patients dying and their not being replaced by others from the community. In the year 1989–90, for example, the long-stay hospital population fell by 2800, but 710 resulted from the deaths of residents, a quarter of the total (Collins, 1992). The people who would once have filled the beds vacated now remain in the community, where they join the queue for support services from the SSDs. Social services departments have to stretch their resources to support the increasing number of people remaining in the community who have special needs.

A national survey conducted in April 1992 of SSD readiness to take on community care changes showed that 66 per cent of authorities were considering or had already decided on organizational changes to accommodate assessment and care management: 81 per cent have planned devolved budgetary systems for use by care managers. Eighty-five per cent of SSDs had made progress towards developing mechanisms for purchasing and commissioning services from private and voluntary agencies, with 16 per cent having made substantial progress. Of the fifty-seven authorities which had reorganized or considered reorganizing to meet the demands of care management and assessment, fourteen were involved in creating a purchaser/provider split, five had created separate adult, children and families divisions, two authorities had done both, and others had introduced care management teams, purchasing teams, locality teams and single door assessment schemes. Nearly the same number had a clear idea of the range and scope of the private and voluntary sector providers likely to be active in their areas post-April 1993.

The Craven Community Care Project in North Yorkshire was funded by the Joseph Rowntree Memorial Trust to evaluate links between statutory and independent sector providers (Henderson, 1992). The study looked at the services provided in the private sector, how owners/managers anticipated future working arrangements with statutory service providers, and whether they foresaw changes in private sector provision. Several identified day care as a growth area, although only one nursing and one residential home planned to expand to include it. There was also resistance towards developing respite care and domiciliary services due to 'anxiety and uncertainty' over funding. Local authorities have powers to inspect residential and nursing homes but none with respect to domiciliary services (as a result of a rejection of a separate Act amendment). It is expected that authorities will make a grant to the cheapest voluntary organization/ private sector provider given tendering arrangements. Some charities are therefore likely to go out of business, and others that obtain contract may supply a lower quality of service – the implication is that charities should become more entrepreneurial to supplement any grant they receive.

The Department of Health intends to issue guidance on charges for domiciliary and day care services as a recent survey has identified a trend towards increased complexity of charging arrangements (House of Commons Health Committee, 1993b). The survey (Balloch, 1993) showed how free home care has dropped by about one-third since 1990 and that there is evidence of further restrictions on eligibility; for example, removal of means-testing through charging a higher rate for those not on income support or housing benefit, plus extending the range of extra charges to clients receiving attendance allowance or the care component of disability living allowance.

Recent research on housing, seen as a cornerstone of community-based services, has highlighted difficulties in partnership arrangements between local authorities and housing agencies (Arnold and Page, 1992). This study revealed limited involvement of housing authorities as partners in community care planning. There were also conflicting perceptions: housing providers saw care practitioners as being unaware of their professional expertise and resource constraints; care agencies saw housing managers as insensitive to community care priorities. At root the new arrangements mean social services and housing must agree roles and responsibilities (Warner, 1992). Housing departments have a significant strategic responsibility to target resources, yet there has been little evidence to visualize at ministerial level the need for strong partnership and to erode funding anomalies and other obstacles. There have been further problems on a national scale relating to the discharge of people from long-stay hospitals. Despite Department of Health (1989c) insistence on the importance of making adequate advance arrangements, the result has been a lack of community support and homelessness for many suffering from psychiatric illness (Stein, 1993). Such people need to be registered with a GP, are likely to be out of touch with a range of services (e.g. the Department of Social Security), and are unlikely to keep up outpatient appointments (Medical Campaign Project, 1990).

The White Paper asserted that 'service providers [should] make practical support for carers a high priority' (Department of Health, 1989a: para. 1.11). Yet much research and local evidence has shown that this has a long way to go (Parker, 1989; Glendinning, 1991; Morris, 1991; Keith, 1992). The legislation offers little basic sustenance to carers, arguably the main service providers (around six million, approximately 14 per cent of British adults). The claim is that '[there are] substantial work related costs incurred by carers with full-time employment; and second, the financial dependency of carers without full-time earnings, on their spouse, sibling or the person being cared for' (Glendinning, 1991).

Studies showing how carers are undervalued and need increased help and support (Wilkin, 1979; Ayer and Alaszewski, 1984; Graham, 1987; Hubert, 1991; Evans et al., 1992) have more recently been paralleled by wider critiques of interventionist policies and services which ignore the experiences of users and carers and the relationships that exist between them (Dalley, 1988; Brown and Smith, 1989; Corbett, 1989; Borsay, 1990; Oliver, 1990). There is a need also for a better partnership between workers and users (Lindow, 1991; Drake, 1992; Kerruish and Reardon, 1992; Marsh and Fisher, 1992), as it has been found, for example, that users often lack information, do not participate in decision-making, complain about not being taken seriously enough and lack the means for empowerment. Marsh and Fisher (1992) identify key areas for partnership-oriented staff development, including the need for explicit organizational commitment, partnership principles, the value of viewing services through users' eyes, and the need to increase the evaluation of training and of practice change.

> 'The challenge is ... to ensure that we provide a seamless service based entirely around the needs and wishes of the users of care and their carers'
>
> (Virginia Bottomley, then Minister of Health,
> Department of Health press release, 1991)

User empowerment and studies of users' views have gathered increasing momentum (Williams and Shoultz, 1982; Crawley, 1988; Whittaker, 1990; Mackie, 1992; Simons, 1992), partly in response to the community care agenda and partly as a result of major dissatisfactions with the quality of many existing services. This literature has demonstrated, among other things, the need for continuity and fruitful relationships with the people who look after them, the need to be listened to, the need (by disabled people) to be treated as ordinary citizens, and the need for more effective resourcing of self-advocacy groups.

A network of local services needs to provide a backdrop to the achievement of keyworker responsibility at the individual user level. If care management (or targeting) is to succeed, then it is important that people are not 'lost' in the community, that the 'new market' is flexible and sufficiently robust to create a broad range of provision. Everything hinges on overall resourcing and management of services at a personal level. A major fear is that the market will create disintegrated provision and that the keyworker system will be spread too thinly. Dant and Gearing (1993), describing the Case Manager Project, demonstrated this advocacy role by showing how the approach depended on the plurality of services and the complexity facing the user: '[The case managers] did not only act like "brokers", merely connecting people to services to meet their needs. The active, advocate role was necessary because services and resources needed to be negotiated, even fought for – and not always successfully ... [suggesting] scarcity and lack of accessibility to people who need them.'

Of central importance is networking involving informal care providers – family, friends and neighbours (Bulmer, 1993). Although individuals or families with problems remain the centre of attention, the focus should be upon individuals within the networks of which they form a part. This connection was emphasized in the Barclay Report on social work: 'Caring networks in a community need to have ready access to statutory and voluntary services and to contribute their experience to decisions on how resources contributed by these services are used within their community' (1982: p. 202). It is hoped that the present government's alleged firm commitment to a policy of community care will succeed in striking this balance as a means of enabling people 'to live as independently as possible in their own homes' (Department of Health, 1989a: para. 1.1).

Overview

This chapter discusses planning leading up to the Community Care Act and some of the principles and strategies embodied in the legislation. It draws out some of the difficulties facing statutory agencies in implementing the reforms, e.g. inadequate commitment to financing, setting out a suitable infrastructure and staffing policy, and the involvement of users. Professional staff now have the job of matching individual needs with the realities of the supply side. The service brokerage and advocacy role are set against a market-style culture propped up by diminishing public resources. In 1992, the government decided to introduce a ringfenced special transitional grant and a further sum to recognize new burdens forced on local authorities as a result of changes to the Independent Living Fund. A precondition of receiving a grant was for local authorities to supply acceptable evidence of joint arrangements, discharge procedures and alliance with the independent sector. Problems still exist over assessing unmet needs, recurring funding and top-up payments arising from discrepancies between benefits and charges.

The argument is made for systematic planning of the workforce of individual purchaser and provider agencies supported by a comprehensive training strategy to emphasize shared/inter-agency training. In areas like assessment and care planning, the evidence shows skills can be transferred among different groups (e.g. residential carers, domiciliary carers, social workers), offering greater flexibility to the care management process. The participation of users and carers remains central to the success of the reforms – participation in planning and delivering services – and probably presents the main challenge to current orthodoxy.

References

Arnold, P. and Page, D. (1992). *Housing and Community Care: Bricks and Mortar or Foundation for Action?* Hull: University of Humberside/Joseph Rowntree Foundation Publications.

Atkinson, I. and McHaffie, H. (1992). Shared cares. *Health Service Journal*, 14 May, pp. 24–5.

Audit Commission (1986). *Making a Reality of Community Care*. London: HMSO.

Audit Commission (1992). *Homeward Bound: A New Course for Community Health*. London: HMSO.

Ayer, S. and Alaszewski, A. (1984). *Community Care and the Mentally Handicapped: Services for Mothers and Their Mentally Handicapped Children*. London: Croom Helm.

Balloch, S. (1993). Charging ahead. *Community Care*, 19 August, p. 17.

Barclay Report (1982). *Social Workers: Their Role and Tasks*. London: Bedford Square Press.

Beardshaw, V. and Towell, D. (1990). *Assessment and Case Management: Implications for the Implementation of 'Caring for People'*. King's Fund Institute Briefing Paper 10. London: King's Fund.

Bell, L. (1993). Home alone. *Community Care*, 25 February, pp. i–ii.

Borsay, A. (1990). Disability and attitudes to family care in Britain: Towards a sociological perspective. *Disability, Handicap and Society*, 5(2): 107–122.

Brown, H. and Smith, H. (1989). Whose 'ordinary life' is it anyway? *Disability, Handicap and Society*, 4(2): 105–120.

Brown, J. (1992). Professional boundaries in mental handicap: A policy analysis of joint training. In Thompson, T. and Mathias, P. (eds), *Standards and Mental Handicap*, pp. 352–70. London: Ballière Tindall.

Bulmer, M. (1993). The social basis of community care. In Bornat, J. *et al.* (eds), *Community Care: A Reader*. Basingstoke: Macmillan/Open University.

Bynoe, I.K. (1993). Rights and duties. *Community Care*, 25 March, pp. ii–iii.

Central Council for Education and Training in Social Work (1989). *Regulations for Programmes Leading to the Diploma in Social Work*. London: CCETSW.

Central Council for Education and Training in Social Work (1992). *Learning Together: Shaping New Services for People with Learning Disabilities*. Developing Partnerships in the Caring Professions 1. London: CCETSW.

Challis, D. (1993). Care management: Observations from a programme of research. *PSSRU Bulletin*, No. 9, July, pp. 33–4.

Cheetham, J. (1991). Community care: Bridging the gaps. *Community Care*, 4 July, pp. 24–5.

Collins, J. (1992). *When the Eagles Fly: A Report on Resettlement of People with Learning Difficulties from Long-stay Institutions*. London: Values into Action, Oxford House, Derbyshire Street.

Common, R. and Flynn, N. (1992). *Contracting for Care.* York: Joseph Rowntree Foundation Publications.

Corbett, J. (1989). The quality of life in the 'independence curriculum'. *Disability, Handicap and Society,* 4(2): 145–64.

Counsel and Care (1991). *Community Care: The Gaps.* London: Counsel and Care for the Elderly.

Crawley, B. (1988). *The Growing Voice: A Survey of Self-advocacy Groups in Adult Training Centres and Hospitals in Great Britain.* London: CMH Publications.

Croft, S. and Beresford, P. (1989). Time for social work to gain new confidence. *Social Work Today,* 13 April, pp. 16–18.

Dalley, G. (1988). *Ideologies of Caring: Rethinking Community and Collectivism.* Basingstoke: Macmillan Education.

Dant, T. and Gearing, B. (1993). Key workers for elderly people in the community. In Bornat, J. *et al.* (eds), *Community Care: A Reader.* Basingstoke: Macmillan/Open University.

Davies, P. (1988). Redefining the roles of community care providers. *Health Service Journal,* 17 March, p. 294.

Department of Health (1989a). *Caring for People: Community Care in the Next Decade and Beyond.* Cm. 849. London: HMSO.

Department of Health (1989b). *Working for Patients.* Cm. 555. London: HMSO.

Department of Health (1989c). Discharge of patients from hospital. *Management,* 5(21): 29.

Department of Health/Social Services Inspectorate (1990). *Caring for People: Joint Training Project (Specification).* London: Department of Health.

Department of Health/Social Services Inspectorate (1991a). *Purchase of Service: Practice Guidance.* London: Department of Health.

Department of Health/Social Services Inspectorate (1991b). *Training for Community Care: A Joint Approach.* London: HMSO.

Department of Health/Social Services Inspectorate/LBTC (1992). *Purchase of Service: Training Guidelines.* Available from LBTC, Training for Care, 9 Tavistock Place, London WC1H 9SN, UK.

Departments of Health and Social Security (1993). *Government Response to the Third Report from the Health Committee Session 1992–93, Community Care: Funding from April 1993.* Cm. 2188. London: HMSO.

District Nursing Association UK (1993). *Nursing Skill Mix in the District Nursing Service: Joint Response from DNA and HVA.* Edinburgh: DNA.

Drake, R. (1992). Consumer participation: The voluntary sector and the concept of power. *Disability, Handicap and Society,* 7(3): 267–78.

Edmonston, J. (1988). Managing the manpower resource: 1. The nature of the problem. *Hospital and Health Services Review,* 15: 37–43.

Evans, G. *et al.* (1992). Observing the delivery of a domiciliary support service. *Disability, Handicap and Society,* 7(1): 19–34.

George, M. (1993). Following the Act. *Community Outlook,* April, pp. 23–4.

Glendinning, C. (1988). The invisible carers. *New Society,* 13 May.

Glendinning, C. (1991). Losing ground: Social policy and disabled people in Great Britain, 1980–90. *Disability, Handicap and Society,* 6(1): 3–20.

Glennerster, H. (1991). The planning process. *Community Care,* 11 July, pp. 20–22.

Gourlay, R. (1991). Re-profiling the labour force. *International Journal of Health Care,* 4(1): 3–6.

Graham, H. (1987). Women's poverty and caring. In Glendinning, C. and Millar, J. (eds), *Women and Poverty in Britain*. Brighton: Wheatsheaf.

Griffiths, R. (1988). *Community Care: Agenda for Action*. A Report to the Secretary of State for Social Services. London: HMSO.

Griffiths, R. (1992). Making it happen. *Community Care*, 23 January, pp. 20–22.

Henderson, J. (1992). Staying private or going public. *Community Care*, 9 July, pp. 24–5.

Hepplewhite, R. (1989). The Griffiths White Paper: Package planned in good faith. *Health Service Journal*, 28 September, p. 1192.

House of Commons Health Committee (1993a). *Third Report, Community Care: Funding from April 1993*, Vol. I. London: HMSO.

House of Commons Health Committee (1993b). *Sixth Report, Community Care: The Way Forward*, Vol. I. London: HMSO.

Hoyes, L. and Means, R. (1993). *User Empowerment and the Reform of Community Care: A Study of Early Implementation in Four Local Authorities*. DQM Working Paper 16. SAUS Publications, Rodney Lodge, Bristol BS8 4EA, UK.

Hubert, J. (1991). A mixed blessing. *Community Care*, 28 February, pp. 18–19.

Hunter, D. and Judge, K. (1988). *Griffiths and Community Care: Meeting the Challenge*. King's Fund Institute Briefing Paper 5. London: King's Fund.

Institute for Health Service Management (1992). *Seamless Service – A Stitch in Time: Care in the Community*. IHSM, 75 Portland Place, London W1N 4AN, UK.

John, K. (1993). *Fit for the Community: A Practical Guide to Care Management and Community Care of People with Mental Health Problems*. Positive Publications, 84 Dowanhill Road, London SE6 1SY, UK.

Keith, L. (1992). Who cares wins? Women, caring and disability. *Disability, Handicap and Society*, 7(2): 167–75.

Kerruish, A. and Reardon, C. (1992). Power sharing. *Health Service Journal*, 23 April, pp. 26–7.

King, J. (1993). Mission accomplished. *Community Care*, 15 April, pp. 18–19.

Knapp, M. (1993). The costing process: Background theory. In Netten, A. and Beecham, J. (eds), *Costing Community Care: Theory and Practice*. Aldershot: PSSRU/Ashgate Publishing.

Knapp, M., Netten, A. and Beecham, J. (1993). Costing community care. In Netten, A. and Beecham, J. (eds), *Costing Community Care: Theory and Practice*. Aldershot: PSSRU/Ashgate Publishing.

Langan, M. (1990). Community care in the 1990s: The community care White Paper, 'Caring for People'. *Critical Social Policy*, 10(2): 59–70.

Lindow, V. (1991). Towards user power. *Health Service Journal*, 101 (5266): 18.

Lunn, T. (1988). Made for each other? *Community Care*, 28 April, pp. 28–30.

MacKenzie, A. (1993). Purchasing excellence. *Community Outlook*, May, p. 14.

Mackie, L. (1992). *Community Care: Users' Experiences*. London: NALGO/Institute for Public Policy Research.

Malin, N. (ed.) (1993a). *Community Care for People with Learning Disabilities*. Report of CCETSW Northern Region Conference Series. Sheffield: School of Health and Community Studies, Sheffield Hallam University.

Malin, N. (1993b). Successful community care requires well trained staff. *Community Living*, 6(4): 20–22.

Malin, N. (1993c). *Staff Training and Community Care*. Department of Health Social Services Inspectorate, 67 Albion Street, Leeds LS1 5AA, UK.

Marsh, P. and Fisher, M. (1992). Do we measure up? *Community Care*, 14 May, pp. 18–19.

Massie, B. (1992). Empty wrappings. Inside: Involving Service Users. *Community Care*, 26 March, pp. i–ii.

Medical Campaign Project (1990). *Good Practice on Discharge of Single Homeless People with Particular Reference to Mental Health Units*. London: Medical Campaign Project.

Mitchell, D. (1993). The training treadmill. *Community Care*, 11 March, pp. 18–19.

Morris, J. (1991). *Pride Against Prejudice: Transforming Attitudes to Disability*. London: Women's Press.

NHSME (1992). *The Nursing Skill Mix in the District Nursing Service*. London: HMSO.

Nolan, M. and Grant, G. (1989). Addressing needs of informal carers: A neglected area of nursing practice. *Journal of Advanced Nursing*, 14, 950–61.

Oldham, C. (1991). *Paying for Care*. York: Joseph Rowntree Foundation Publications.

Oliver, M. (1990). *The Politics of Disablement*. Basingstoke: Macmillan.

Parker, G. (1989). The same difference? The experience of men and women caring for a spouse with a disability or chronic illness. Paper presented at the *Social Policy Association Conference*, University of Bath, July.

Phillips, M. (1989). How will it be after Griffiths? *Social Work Today*, 28 September, p. 20.

Schofield, S. (1992). Bradford Social Services Training Plan. City of Bradford Metropolitan Council.

Simons, K. (1992). *Sticking Up for Yourself*. York: Joseph Rowntree Foundation Publications.

Stein, T. (1993). The long goodbye. *Health Service Journal*, 11 March, pp. 28–9.

Teasdale, K. (1993). The case for change: Implications of the 'Caring for People' White Paper. *Professional Nurse*, May, pp. 543–5.

Thompson, T. and Mathias, P. (1992). *Standards and Mental Handicap: Keys to Competence*. London: Ballière Tindall.

Todd, M. (1993). Education and training. In Brigden, P. and Todd, M. (eds), *Concepts in Community Care for People with a Learning Difficulty*. Basingstoke: Macmillan.

Ward, I. (1990). A programme for change: Current issues in services for people with learning difficulties. In Booth, T. (ed.), *Better Lives*. Social Services Monographs: Research in Practice. Sheffield: Joint Unit for Social Services Research, University of Sheffield.

Warner, N. (1992). Housing discontent. *Community Care*, 4 June, p. 14.

Whittaker, A. (1990). *How are Self-advocacy Groups Developing? An Informal Survey of Groups of People with Learning Difficulties*. London: King's Fund.

Wilkin, D. (1979). *Caring for the Mentally Handicapped Child*. London: Croom Helm.

Williams, P. and Shoultz, B. (1982). *We Can Speak For Ourselves*. London: Souvenir Press.

Wistow, G. (1993). Community care plans: A strategic overview. In Malin, N. (ed.), *Community Care for People with Learning Disabilities*. Report of CCETSW Northern Region Conference Series. Sheffield: School of Health and Community Studies, Sheffield Hallam University.

2 Management and finance

Bob Hudson

The funding issue is at the heart of the new approach to community care. Arguably the main imperative behind both the Griffiths Report (1988) and the community care White Paper *Caring for People* (Department of Health 1989a) was the need to halt the open-ended social security subsidy to independent residential and nursing homes. However, although a political consensus seems to have gathered around the new system, the funding issue again seems likely to overshadow the changes and prejudice the effectiveness of them. This chapter explores the funding dilemma. It gives an account of the nature and scale of expenditure on community care, examines the argument that there is a 'funding crisis' and considers some of the implications of this for service entitlement.

Community care: The nature and scale of expenditure

A broad definition of community care encompassing the activities of social services authorities, health authorities and social security, reveals that expenditure almost doubled in real terms in the 1980s (see Fig. 1). A narrower perspective on community care focuses upon the activities of local authority social services departments (SSDs), who will be the 'lead agents' in the post-1993 setting. Here also, the increase in expenditure over the past decade or so seems substantial, though the precise scale of the rise is contentious. The Annual Report of the Department of Health (1990–91) showed that net current expenditure on local authority personal social services (PSS) had increased by 52 per cent in real terms between 1978–89 and 1990–91, but that this fell to 22.3 per cent after allowing for pay and price increases in the personal social services field. This represents a more modest average annual increase in gross current spending of 2.3 per cent. In 1989–90, total net expenditure in the UK was £4.7 billion (around £80 per head of total population), and Table 1 gives more detailed figures for England showing the difference between gross and net expenditure before and after deducting income from charges.

Figure 1 Expenditure on adult community care (from Audit Commission, 1992).

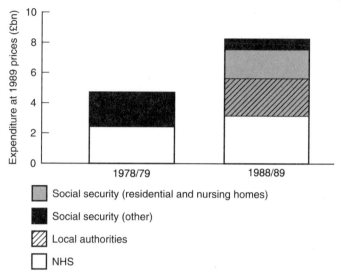

Social security (residential and nursing homes)

Social security (other)

Local authorities

NHS

Note: Social Security (other) includes mobility, invalid care, severe disability and attendance allowances.

Table 1 Personal social services in England, 1989–90 (£billion)

Current expenditure	Gross	4.2
	Charges	0.5
	Net	3.7
Capital	Gross	0.2
	Income	0.1
	Net	0.1
Total	Gross	4.4
	Income	0.6
	Net	3.8

Source: HM Treasury (1991)

Estimates of expenditure on different groups of users are important, because much PSS spending goes on children's services which are not always included as 'community care' activities. Using data from the Department of Health and the Chartered Institute of Public Finance Accountants, Hulme (1991) produced an estimate for England for 1989–90 (Table 2).

Obtaining a clear picture of local activity is further compounded by the spending variations between local authorities. Pressures on services are

Table 2 PSS expenditure by user group in England, 1989–90

	% of total	£bn	£ per head
Children	32	1.2	26
Elderly	45	1.7	36
Physically handicapped	7	0.3	6
Mentally handicapped	14	0.5	11
Mentally ill	2	0.1	

unlikely to bear equally between authorities, and under current arrangements it is up to individual authorities to make judgements about the allocation of resources between services in the light of local assessments of need and priorities. However, the Select Committee on Health (House of Commons Health Committee, 1991) looked at figures for the period 1984–85 to 1990–91 and found variations in spending between individual authorities, ranging from growth in excess of 40 per cent to reductions in excess of 5 per cent, and expressed concern about the relationship between spending levels and service needs. This concern has been echoed by the Social Services Policy Forum (1992), which described access to services as 'a game of geographical chance' and criticized the way in which local autonomy on resource allocation has taken precedence over equal access to services.

It is, however, necessary to go beyond PSS spending to get a proper picture of the development of community care activity. In particular, the need to control the growth in social security spending on independent residential and nursing homes was a principal target of the community care legislation. In December 1979, the level of supplementary benefit paid to people in such homes stood at £10 million nationally (12 000 claimants); after the April 1991 benefit upratings, the level of income support was estimated to be £1625 million (220 000 claimants). Despite the government's efforts to control spending on these benefits, the amount paid out continued to rise dramatically, and the decision to keep the subsidy arrangements in force until April 1993 is likely to have increased the amount to around £2000 million.

Such availability inevitably encouraged both health and local authorities to make their community care programmes 'social security efficient', and the perversity of this in relation to home-based care was well emphasized by the seminal Audit Commission report of 1986. Accordingly, when the government's proposals for a new structure for providing community care were announced in the 1989 White Paper, one of the main planks was a new way of funding community care. Paragraphs 17–18 laid out the intentions:

The Government proposes to introduce a single unified budget to cover the cost of social care, whether in a person's own home or in a residential care or nursing home. The new budget will include the care element of social security payments to people in private and voluntary, residential care and nursing homes. Local authorities are to be given responsibility for managing this budget and making best use of funds available in the light of an assessment of an individual's needs . . . People who enter homes under the new funding structure and who need public financial support will no longer have their care costs met by social security. In place of the special limits they will be able to claim help from the normal Income Support system of personal allowances and premiums, and from Housing Benefit. They will receive assistance on the same basis as that which they could obtain in their own homes. The financial incentive towards residential care under present Income Support rules will therefore be eliminated.

(Department of Health, 1989a: paras 17–18)

Although this may well provide a solution to the government's problem (by capping the social security subsidy and transferring responsibility for it to local authorities), it is far from clear that this will leave local authorities in a position to develop and fund an adequate community care strategy. Indeed, it may simply lead to a crisis in community care funding.

A crisis in community care funding?

The world of community care in the 1990s seems beset by paradox. On the one hand, there has been a broad professional and political welcome for many components of the changes, especially community care planning, care management, closer collaboration between welfare agencies and some notion of user involvement. On the other hand, it is clear that these cannot be cost-free ventures, and there seems to be little confidence that they will be properly funded. To get a better understanding of the funding issue, four broad areas will be examined: the growing demand for support; the curtailment of local authority autonomy; funding in the post-1993 scenario; and the wider constraints arising from economic recession.

A growing demand for personal care?

Although it is generally acknowledged that the demand for personal care will increase, Hulme (1991) suggested several factors which may partly diminish the pressure:

• Demographic pressures promise to be slightly less in the first half of the 1990s than the second half of the 1980s – the growth of personal social services required to match the growing number of elderly people is estimated at 0.8 per cent per annum rather than the current 1.2 per cent.

• As the income of elderly people increases from retirement pensions and asset sales, more will be able to contribute to the cost of services or buy from the private sector.
• There are possibilities of efficiency gains through the control of costs and better targeting through care management. This may be an optimistic suggestion, since the new assessment procedures could just as easily uncover greater unmet need.

The House of Commons Health Committee (1991) found the Department of Health to be evasive and equivocal about the relationship between a specific growth rate for PSS and changes in levels of potential demand. Although conceding in an earlier memorandum to the committee that it used an estimate of demographic and similar pressures of 2 per cent per annum, the department subsequently denied the use of such a benchmark, arguing that only the demographic element is precisely calculable and the rest is a much more general assessment. Notwithstanding any estimates of unmet need which may emerge from the new planning and assessment systems, there is already convincing evidence of substantial shortfall. For example, the OPCS survey of disabled people in the late 1980s (Martin *et al.*, 1988) showed that only a small proportion of the one million adults needing help with self-care activities got it from the formal services – of the 80 000 who needed a lot of help both day and night, only 28 per cent were getting it from services.

The curtailment of local financial autonomy

Since 1981, the government has been fixated with the scale of local government spending, even though its growth has not been out of line with the growth of the economy as a whole. Three strategies have been adopted to constrict local spending: a consistent reduction in the proportion of local expenditure funded by government grant from 60 per cent in 1979 to 42 per cent in 1990–91, with a corresponding increase in the contribution from householders, up from 17 to 28 per cent; an increase in the cost to local residents of an extra £1 expenditure, achieved by reducing the government subsidy for 'extra' local authority spending; and, if all else fails, by rate capping and poll tax capping. Indeed, in 1992–93, poll tax capping was extended to councils with budgets under £15 million, with fifty local councils having to peg spending or make cuts in their budgets.

These strong-arm tactics have made it difficult to improve community services, but the increase in demand for such provision, coupled with the unpopularity of the poll tax, resulted in a £3.7 billion poll tax subsidy in April 1990, followed by a £4.3 billion subsidy in the March 1991 budget.

The effect of this was to cut £140 from poll tax bills and deliver a substantial defeat to the Treasury in its attempt to control local spending, but it failed to usher in the 1990 NHS and Community Care Act. The main reason for the postponement of the community care reforms from April 1991 until April 1993 was the need to limit the political damage thought likely to result from an additional £15 on the average poll tax bill. Since then, there has been some evidence of a tighter retrenchment. In a recent survey, Hatchett (1992) reported the majority of English and Welsh SSDs to be facing substantial cuts in 1992–93. Typical cost-cutting measures reported are the closure or transfer to trust status of residential homes, the closure of day centres, the introduction of or increase in charges for home helps, and reductions in transport and other services for disabled people.

A good part of the problem for local authorities is the way in which central government calculates its spending requirements on social care services. The standard spending assessment (SSA) is the amount the government calculates local councils should spend to deliver a standard service each year. It acts not simply as a distributional tool, but is used to decide which authorities should be 'capped' – a fate which befell twenty-one councils in 1990, seventeen in 1991 and fifty in 1992. In such circumstances, the fairness of the procedure used to calculate the SSA is critical. Broadly, SSA calculations for the personal social services are based upon three rather crude categories: elderly people (accounting for some 45 per cent of the calculated expenditure), children (35 per cent) and 'other' (20 per cent). In the case of elderly people, the main weighting is given to the simple global number, all of whom are seen as potential service users. This could be said to favour southern shire counties, which contain a lot of relatively wealthy elderly people who are less likely to use local authority services. Again, the formula contains no assessment of the numbers of people with a mental illness, learning disability or physical disability in a given area, nor does it take into account a range of 'environmental' factors such as housing conditions. In short, the SSA does not make a sophisticated attempt to measure need.

It is easy to see why some local authorities regard 'overspending' as arising from errors in SSA calculation, rather than from fiscal profligacy. In 1990, for example, capping came into force if local authorities spent either 12.5 per cent more than their SSA or £75 per head more than projected by the SSA. However, in inner London, social services spending was 17 per cent greater than their SSAs, and most metropolitan authorities were spending above their 'limit'. Hatchett (1992) found that in 1992–93, ten social services authorities faced capping, but 64 per cent had budgets above their SSA, with an average difference of almost £6 million. The switch from the poll tax to the council tax will not bring about any changes to the SSA position.

Funding residential and nursing home care after April 1993

From April 1993, responsibility for funding residential and nursing home care (over and above normal social security entitlements) will fall to social services authorities who will have transferred to them from the Department of Social Security a budget thought to be sufficient for this purpose. The size and scope of this budget has been described by the Social Security Select Committee (1991) as determining the success of the whole of the government's community care plans.

There are two components in this transfer. First, the transfer of Income Support monies to local authorities to enable them to fund the 'care' element of the new unified budget. The calculation of the amount to be transferred has had to take account of four factors: the Income Support that would have been payable under the pre-April 1993 scheme; normal Income Support and housing benefit payable to new residents; the continuing commitment to those residents with preserved rights to the pre-1993 scheme; and the rate at which local authorities will assume responsibility for the care of new clients. The second main component concerns the calculation of housing benefit entitlement to cover the 'rent' costs of accommodation. It would be administratively problematic for a housing benefit authority to be put in the position of trying to assess a 'reasonable rent' for every room in every establishment, yet if the assessment formula is too broad, it may lead to a shortfall in funding for residents.

One of the reasons for delaying the implementation of the community care reforms for two years until April 1993 was the inability of the main central government departments (the Departments of Social Security and Health) to come to an agreement on this transfer, either between themselves or with the local authority associations. There are disagreements on several fronts: the rate at which the number of existing 'protected' residents will decline; the demand for new placements (the government estimate is 25 000 per annum compared with the 45 000 of the local authority associations); the formula for distribution between local authorities (e.g. the proposal to divert money to those authorities with the most independent homes is less sophisticated than weighting the formula to favour those authorities with the most residents in receipt of Income Support).

However, the most politically contentious issue is the estimated shortfall between fees payable and actual costs. The Association of Metropolitan Authorities estimated the shortfall to amount to £935 million in 1993–94, but the government refused to include in the transferred amount a sum to cover any such gap. The danger of such a position was highlighted in 1990 by the Social Services Select Committee (1990b):

> If current benefits are insufficient to meet the costs of care, the sums transferred to local authorities from social security benefits will be insufficient to meet their costs of purchasing residential care . . . If

the transfer of money to local authorities is not adequate, the new system will begin in deficit with inadequate resources to fund existing needs, let alone develop new services.

The advice from the Department of Health to local authorities is that they should use their purchasing muscle to force down the fees of home owners, but an equally likely possibility is that local authorities find themselves dealing with cartels of homeowners maintaining or forcing up prices. This in turn might lead to a pronounced push towards domiciliary care (one of the key objectives of the White Paper), leading to a drop in the occupancy rates of homes, an increase in unit costs and little or no savings. This in turn raises the possibility of evictions and home closures. The Social Security Select Committee (1991) could find only anecdotal evidence of home closure, but in evidence to the committee, both the Association of Metropolitan Authorities and the National Association of Citizens Advice Bureaux reported instances of people being asked to move to less expensive homes. The April 1993 changes will in any case reshape the position to the disadvantage of pre-April 1993 residents. From 1993, where local authorities have assessed a user as in need of residential care, they will be required to meet the full cost of it, whereas prior residents will have no such entitlement. Relatives and charities 'topping up' the fees of pre-1993 residents will continue to do so.

One of the difficulties with this issue is the lack of real information about the difference between the sums being paid out in Income Support and the sums people are actually paying to homes. The Department of Social Security commissioned a survey of the running costs in residential and nursing homes (Price Waterhouse, 1990), which concluded that nationally, median costs were at or only slightly above Income Support rates in residential homes, but were above Income Support rates by a similar margin in nursing homes. These findings were hotly disputed, particularly on the grounds that no attempt had been made to relate costs to measures of quality of care or of the dependency level of residents. What is not in doubt is that relatives and charities have been increasingly called upon to meet the cost-fee gap. A survey of 117 charities (Wright, 1992) came up with several important findings: between them the charities spent around £5 million on topping-up the Income Support of 6772 elderly people; the charities themselves had an average income deficit of 16.8 per cent in 1991–92; the average fee shortfall in 1991 among elderly people approaching the charities for help was £57 per week; and the topping-up activities absorbed 38 per cent of the charities' expenditure on elderly people as a whole.

In their review of the issue, Henwood and Wistow (1991) suggested that these inadequate benefit levels can have a number of consequences for individuals and their families: a minimal or non-existent choice of home;

Table 3 Special transitional grant in England (£million)

Year	DSS transfer	Infrastructure grant
1993–94	399	140
1994–95	651	Not given
1995–96	518	Not given

a two-tier system of care in which Income Support residents are required to share a room; the running down of an individual's capital reserves, which may result in a carer losing the home; the use of a resident's personal allowances to meet the fee shortfall; families and friends feeling obliged to meet the shortfall; increasing pressures on charitable resources to contribute towards care costs; pressures to move to a cheaper home within the independent sector; and an enforced removal to a local authority home or long-stay hospital care, if these facilities are still in existence. A further consequence is that in order to balance their budgets, local authorities may raise charges for services without due regard for ability to pay, and at a time of increasing impoverishment among those groups who need to use the services (Balloch, 1991).

Eventually, in October 1992, the Department of Health revealed the amount of money SSDs were to receive to begin implementation of the community care changes in the following April. A distinction was drawn between the monies transferred from the Department of Social Security and an 'infrastructure' grant to develop information systems, care management and so forth. Together these elements were termed the 'Special Transitional Grant' and the amounts involved are shown in Table 3. This money will be given a degree of protection in that each annual amount will be 'ringfenced' for that year, though the cumulative total will not be ringfenced. Even this is a significant policy change, for the government had consistently set its face against the very principle of ringfencing prior to the funding announcement. The Special Transitional Grant (STG) will be phased out in its fourth year, with all monies then being allocated under the traditional SSA formula.

Disputation immediately arose over the adequacy of these amounts, particularly over whether they matched the estimated numbers of elderly and disabled people likely to require assessments under the new arrangements. Department of Health funding is based upon an estimate of 110 000 people coming forward for care in 1993–94 – an underestimate of 12 000 according to the local authority associations, who sought 1993–94 funding of £634 million in social security transfers and £194 million in start-up costs. Based on these figures, the shortfall for 1993–94 alone will be £289 million, though the truth probably is that most local authorities had no accurate estimate of the cost implications of the changes.

Much less attention has been given to a further aspect of the funding – the attachment of conditions to the ringfencing arrangements. Some of these have been well-received. For example, all local authorities were required to have in place by the end of 1992 agreed strategies with health authorities for placing people in nursing homes and for integrating discharge arrangements with new assessment arrangements. Reaching agreement on such strategies is not the same as having the funding to meet identified needs, but nevertheless the principle of encouraging collaboration by financial penalty may have something to commend it. However, two further conditions – distributional and purchasing – are more problematic.

The view of the Department of Health is that to distribute the social security transfer according to the SSA formula, rather than according to the current location of private homes, would lead to instability for private homeowners who may find local authorities withdrawing residents back to their home areas. The compromise is one whereby half of the transfer is based upon the SSA and half upon current Department of Social Security spending locations. The metropolitan authorities will suffer under this formula, for they tend to be big 'exporters' of residents and may not be funded for this activity.

The purchasing condition is potentially more devastating. The Department of Health initially required local authorities to spend at least 75 per cent of their STG on services provided by the independent sector, with an obligation to demonstrate that their total net expenditure on independent sector providers for 1993–94 had risen by at least the value of 75 per cent of the STG compared with the 1992–93 equivalent. This was a timely reminder that the community care reforms are based upon a New Right ideology and do not warrant the all-party consensus which seems to have arisen.

There are two difficulties with the purchasing condition. First, it disadvantages those authorities whose social security transfer money constitutes less than 75 per cent of their total STG, for in such circumstances the rules will compel them to spend their limited 'infrastructure' money on purchasing possibly unnecessary private care. Most local authorities would have been caught in this trap, with the inner London boroughs most badly affected. This difficulty belatedly dawned upon the Department of Health, which soon removed the £140 million infrastructure money from the purchasing conditions, thereby reducing the independent sector slice of the transferred budget to 62 per cent.

The second difficulty is that many authorities will have no private provision in their area other than residential and nursing home provision. Although one of the key objectives of *Caring for People* (Department of Health, 1989a) is to control the growth of institutional provision and encourage the growth of domiciliary and day care, the latter is not widely available and may not easily flourish. In effect, the '62 per cent rule' will force local authorities to purchase whatever independent care happens to be available and the outcome may well be a further growth in institutional provision.

Community care: The wider economic context

If the ambitious community care reforms are to succeed, then the government will need to honour its commitment to provide proper funding, yet the prospects of this happening seem remote. The world of community care could not expect to be untouched by an economy in which output is falling in all sectors and every region, retail sales are falling, factories closing and unemployment rising. The Public Sector Borrowing Requirement (PSBR) is projected to increase from £13.75 billion (1991–92) to £28 billion (1992–93) and £50 billion (1993–94), and even that is only after adding in substantial privatization proceeds. The culprit is not so much an overshoot in public spending as a growing shortfall in tax revenues, which are down more than £4 billion on projections – corporation tax down £1.1 billion, income tax down £1.8 billion and VAT down £2.2 billion. By July 1992, the government decided to seek huge cuts in planned public spending over the following three years. For 1992–93, the spending target of £244.5 billion was kept, but this meant cuts in some programmes to compensate for an overshoot in social security payments. There are planned reductions totalling £16 billion in the following two years, and this will be unattainable without across-the-board cuts.

It is important to lay out this broader context, for it constitutes the backcloth to the difficult negotiations which the Department of Health will have to conduct with the Treasury to secure adequate funding for the community care reforms. Given the scale of the problem and the political insignificance of community care, it is easy to see how a case can be made out to suggest that the world of community care is facing a 'crisis of funding'. However, there is no economic inevitability about underfunding, for Britain remains a prosperous nation well able to find significant sums of money for political priorities. Since 1979, for example, the richest 5 per cent of the population have received tax reductions representing an annual loss to the Treasury of £12.5 billion, and during the Gulf War the government borrowed somewhere between 0.5 per cent and 1.5 per cent of gross domestic product.

Funding and the reshaping of service entitlements

Although social services authorities have been given lead responsibility for assessing and purchasing social care after April 1993, there remains organizational and financial fragmentation between agencies, with a particular confusion over the boundary between health and social care. Much of the difficulty relates to the use of social security payments over the past decade to covertly redefine entitlements to free health care (Henwood and Wistow, 1991; Henwood, 1992). One of the major reasons for the growth in the number of independent homes is that health authorities have been phasing out their own long-stay beds. Between 1978 and 1988, the number of NHS geriatric beds fell from 58 000 to 53 000, and the pace of decline increased to 5.8 per cent in 1990–91. Instead, increased reliance has been placed upon independent nursing home care, with the Registered Nursing Homes Association calculating that by 1993 its members would cover 46 706 beds, compared with 45 000 in the National Health Service (NHS).

Henwood and Wistow (1991) emphasize that the underlying issue is not so much about who provides care or where it is received, but about the entitlement of individuals to a comprehensive range of free health services. People receiving long-term care from the NHS are entitled to such care at no charge to themselves or their relatives, and have (at least in principle) a similar entitlement to a full range of ancillary services. By contrast, residents in the independent sector may not only be called upon to top up the costs of their care, but may also find themselves paying for support services. A survey by the Association of Directors of Social Services (1992) reported charges for incontinence aids, chiropody, dressings and physiotherapy, all of which people would receive without charge if they were living in their own homes or in NHS hospitals. Some see this as legitimate. In evidence to the Social Security Select Committee (1991), the Chairman of the Nursing Homes Advisory Group of the National Association of Hospital Authorities and Trusts said that nursing home care was not a function of the NHS, a view described by the committee as 'extraordinary'.

All of this would seem to be contrary to NHS guidance. Department of Health (1989b) guidance on discharge from hospital is explicit:

> Where a person moves from hospital to a private nursing home, it should be made quite clear to him/her in writing before the transfer, whether or not the health authority will pay the fees under a contractual arrangement. No NHS patient should be placed in a private nursing or residential care home against his/her wishes if it means that he/she or a relative will be personally responsible for the home's charges.

The Social Security Select Committee (1991) felt:

> there must be doubts about how strictly this guidance is applied ... evidence indicates that in many cases the DoH circular is being disregarded and patients are given no information about the circumstances under which they should continue to be cared for as NHS

patients, whether in hospital or a nursing home. Indeed, patients with significant continuing nursing needs are led to believe that they and their families are responsible for paying for or providing any subsequent care.

The committee went on to suggest that: '. . . in some parts of the NHS, the culture seems to be that nursing home care no longer counts as health care'. Such a view will have been reinforced by a 1991 executive letter from the Department of Health to authorities which sought to draw a distinction between nursing home care provided to those discharged from hospital, and nursing home care for those who require it because of 'continuing ill-health', and which health authorities may fund. The Social Security Committee (1991) found this to be an untenable distinction: 'This is a distinction without a difference, and while it may seem appropriate to those in charge of health authority budgets, it makes little sense for those who need the care'.

The social security subsidy to independent care homes is an example of what can happen when change takes place in an *ad hoc* way – no overt decision was made to phase out geriatric wards, for the practice simply grew as health authorities saw the opportunity to transfer the costs to the budget of another department. A shift to nursing homes could be justified as an attempt to establish more homely and less institutional nursing care for long-term patients, but the expansion has not occurred under contractual arrangements to ensure that specified benefits were being secured. In effect, there has been a dual unplanned shift of funding responsibility from the NHS to the social security system, and from the NHS to individuals and families forced to make good the inadequacies of Income Support. After April 1993, the NHS can still have contractual beds for nursing homes, can still invest in housing for discharged patients and can still make money available via joint finance and dowry payments, but this would seem to require a change in attitude on the part of the National Health Service Management Executive towards continuing care (Westland, 1992).

Conclusion

This chapter has reviewed some of the issues relating to the funding of community care both before and after the April 1993 changes. Several problems have been identified: the relatively modest increase in local authority spending in relation to the growing demands for personal support; the curtailment of local authority autonomy to respond to locally identified need; the more general impact of an economy in recession; the distorting influence of independent homes both in relation to overall funding and to the loss of entitlement to NHS care. It has been argued that there is little prospect of adequate funding for the changes brought in under the NHS and Community Care Act 1990, and that financial blight will inescapably cast a shadow over those many parts of the changes which have secured political, professional and user support.

References

Association of Directors of Social Services (1992). *Private Residential Care in England and Wales*. London: ADSS.

Audit Commission (1986). *Making a Reality of Community Care*. London: HMSO.

Audit Commission (1992). *The Community Revolution*. London: HMSO.

Balloch, S. (1991). Local authority charging policies. *Benefits*, October/November, pp. 40–41.

Department of Health (1989a). *Caring for People: Community Care in the Next Decade and Beyond*. Cm. 849. London: HMSO.

Department of Health (1989b). Discharge of patients from hospital. DoH Circular HC(89)5.

Griffiths, R. (1988). *Community Care: An Agenda for Action*. A Report to the Secretary of State for Social Services. London: HMSO.

Hatchett, W. (1992). Charting the swing of the axe. *Community Care*, 21 May, pp. 8–19.

Henwood, M. (1992). *Through a Glass Darkly: Community Care and Elderly People*. London: King's Fund.

Henwood, M. and Wistow, G. (1991). *Memorandum to Social Security Select Committee, Appendix 15*. London: HMSO.

HM Treasury (1991). *Public Expenditure White Paper*. Cm. 1021. London: HMSO.

House of Commons Health Committee (1991). *Third Report, Session 1990–91, Public Expenditure on Health and Personal Social Services*. London: HMSO.

Hulme, G. (1991). Expenditure on personal social services in the 1980s and 1990s. *Public Money and Management*, Winter, pp. 31–4.

Martin, J., Meltzer, H. and Elliot, D. (1988). *The Prevalence of Disability Amongst Adults*. London: HMSO.

Price Waterhouse (1990). *A Survey of Residential Care and Nursing Home Running Costs*. London: Price Waterhouse.

Social Security Select Committee (1991). *Fourth Report, Session 1990–91, The Financing of Private Residential and Nursing Home Fees*. London: HMSO.

Social Services Policy Forum (1992). *Great Expectations . . . and Spending on Social Services*. London: National Institute for Social Work.

Social Services Select Committee (1990b). *Second Report, Session 1989–90, Community Care: Future Funding of Private and Voluntary Residential Care*. London: HMSO.

Westland, P. (1992). The algebra of mandarins. *Community Care*, 18 June, pp. 20–21.

Wright, F. (1992). *Fee Shortfalls in Residential and Nursing Homes: The Impact on the Voluntary Sector*. Institute of Gerontology. London.

3 Community care planning

Gerald Wistow and Brian Hardy

Introduction

The White Paper *Caring for People* (Department of Health, 1989) was a seminal document in its explicit statement of community care objectives, its recasting of the role of social services departments (SSDs) and its promotion of a mixed economy. Perhaps its most fundamental contribution, however, was to place the identification of need at the centre of management and service delivery processes and to institute, as a statutory requirement, the preparation of a community care plan based on information about community and individual needs. This endorsement of needs-based social planning was all the more remarkable from a government whose scepticism about such activities had been reflected in the abolition, within months of its election in 1979, of the previous national planning system for the personal social services.

In this chapter, we outline the planning framework introduced in the wake of the White Paper, the subsequent NHS and Community Care Act of 1990 and subsequent policy guidance (Department of Health, 1990). We also review early progress in planning, based on an analysis of the first plans published in April 1992, and consider the issues raised by this analysis. Before addressing such matters, however, it is important to understand the context from which the requirement to produce such plans had emerged, including their antecedents in previous planning systems.

Previous community care planning systems

National frameworks for community care planning can be traced back to the early 1960s, with the introduction in 1962, by the Ministry of Health, of ten-year plans for hospital services and the following year for local authority community health and welfare services (Ministry of Health, 1962, 1963). In the latter, local authorities were asked to outline future developments 'without guidance on likely resource trends or on preferred patterns of service provision'. In contrast to this essentially *laissez-faire* approach, the next ten-year planning system was much more interventionist (Webb and Wistow, 1986: 87). Introduced by the Department of Health and Social Security in 1972, this system was based on assumed rates of growth of 10 per cent per annum and a framework of service guidelines, specifying, on a per capita basis, levels of provision for the main services.

This planning system, together with its resource assumptions, rapidly collapsed under the economic pressures produced by the 1973 Arab–Israeli War and attendant oil crisis. However, these pressures in turn emphasized the need to secure the most effective use of available resources. The 1972 ten-year planning system had been intended to secure precisely this end with health and local authorities drawing their plans 'into relationship with one another' and with central and local government regularly reviewing service developments and resource usage (DHSS, 1972). It was, therefore, not surprising that in the mid-1970s the government devised new planning guidelines and systems aimed at integration across the health and personal social services systems. Thus the publication of the consultation document *Priorities for Health and Personal Social Services* (DHSS, 1976) was seen to mark 'the first attempt to establish a single, coherent set of priorities across both sets of services and to express them in terms of quantified targets to be achieved within specified timescales' (Wistow and Henwood, 1989). Based on a new national programme budget, the document specified annual growth rates for particular client groups and services for the period up to 1980 and provided a set of planning 'norms' or guideline levels of service provision.

A new national planning system for the National Health Service (NHS) was also introduced in 1976 and in the following year new arrangements were introduced for planning in the personal social services. These Local Authority Planning Statements (LAPS) differed from the earlier planning system in two important respects. First, the planning horizon was three years not ten; second, the growth assumption was 2 rather than 10 per cent. Common to both systems, however, were the centrally determined planning guidelines or norms. In the case of services to the elderly, for example, the guidelines were for twenty-five residential places, three to four day centre places, twelve home helps and 200 meals a week per thousand population aged sixty-five and over.

Three main characteristics of these planning guidelines should be highlighted:

(i)   they were expressed as levels of service production (inputs and intermediate outputs) rather than as outcomes for users;

(ii) while acting as proxies for need and thus tending to discourage local analysis of the level and structure of need, the guidelines

themselves were apparently derived more from 'best professional judgement' than analysis;
(iii) they focused attention on a relatively narrow range and mix of service options, thereby discouraging innovation and the more flexible use of resources.

(Wistow, 1990)

Thus the national planning systems developed in the 1970s tended to encourage the production of a relatively narrow range of standardized services. They also provided little incentive for local authorities either to analyse need systematically or to experiment with different service mixes, since the guidelines effectively specified 'approved' levels and mixes of provision. It was thus easy for at least some local authorities to equate planning with meeting these service targets, rather than to see it as a continuous process of objective setting, needs mapping, service production and review. In effect, therefore, the planning systems proved more effective as a means of transmitting statistical data to the centre than promoting the development of strategic planning and review functions locally. However, while local authorities tended to view planning as primarily meeting the information needs of the centre, the Conservative government elected in 1979 had little sympathy for its planning inheritance. Thus LAPS was seen to represent an unduly 'detailed, bureaucratic and dirigiste style of planning' (Wistow, 1990: para 2.7). The 1979–80 planning round was cancelled in the wake of spending cuts proposed for the personal social services and LAPS was never resurrected (Webb and Wistow, 1982, 1986).

Significantly, the inadequacies of arrangements for health and social care planning were among the principal issues identified from the mid-1980s in a series of highly critical reports about the implementation of community care (see especially House of Commons Social Services Committee, 1985; Audit Commission, 1986; National Audit Office, 1987; Griffiths, 1988). The last of these reports had been commissioned by the Secretary of State from Sir Roy Griffiths in response to the Audit Commission's critique of the policy contradictions and perverse incentives which, it argued, prevented the effective implementation of community care objectives. Griffiths' report was blunt in its criticism of planning, or rather, the lack of it. There was, he argued, 'only limited evidence of systematic planning' in social services departments (Griffiths, 1988: para. 4.8). Moreover, he concluded that the lack of information and financial management systems at either central or local level 'would plunge most organisations in the private sector into a quick and merciful liquidation' (ibid.: para. 28). At the same time, he was critical of local planning arrangements between health and local authorities, effectively dismissing them as a 'discredited refuge of imploring collaboration and exhorting action' (ibid.: para. 27).

Against this background, the establishment of a community care planning system was inevitably among the 'keystones' of his recommendations. Indeed, the allocation of resources from the centre via a specific grant was to be conditional on the preparation of such an annual plan by social services authorities (Griffiths, 1988: para. 6.35). Payment of the grant would depend on the plans providing evidence of, *inter alia*, the existence of systems for joint planning and action; the adequacy of management systems; the involvement and support of the voluntary sector; costed programmes and timetables for implementation; proposals well-thought out in relation to local needs; value for money; and the development of an enabling role by social services authorities (ibid.: paras 6.35–6.36).

From one perspective, these proposals amounted to a new framework for central–local relations. As such, they effectively took on board the National Audit Office's (1987: para. 5) earlier criticism that, while the NHS review process enabled central government to monitor the progress of health authorities in the development and implementation of community care policies, the Department of Health was unable to review local authority performance in an analogous way (ibid.: para. 5, p. 2). What Griffiths was proposing, therefore, was a planning process which went some considerable way towards meeting the need for what the National Audit Office had termed 'direct and equal oversight' by the centre over both services (ibid.: para. 6). Thus, the linking of resource allocation to the submission of plans prepared in a collaborative context, must in part be seen as an attempt to design accountability and control processes which could secure concerted action at the local level consistent with national policy objectives and priorities.

The Griffiths framework was, however, by no means a mechanism purely for combining what might be termed control downwards with accountability upwards. It also contained a strong localist element within its conception of the planning task. Local plans were to be shaped not only by national policies, as articulated by the Minister for Community Care, but also by a much more systematic analysis of local needs built up at both the local authority and individual levels. Indeed, Griffiths' advocacy of a lead role for local government was strongly based on his belief that elected local authorities were best placed to 'assess local needs, set local priorities, and monitor local performance' (Griffiths, 1988: para. 5.2). At the same time, the community care grant was to be distributed on the basis of a formula which took account of local variations in need.

It is, however, important to emphasize that Griffiths was not solely concerned with managerial structures and improved accountability. His approach not only meant that service delivery should be tailored to individual needs (rather than the latter being accommodated within whatever happened to be existing service patterns), it also implied the availability of an increasing range of service options and service providers. The implication for the planning task was, therefore, the importance of coordination across a wider range of local statutory agencies. Beyond this, Griffiths' proposal for a planned growth in non-statutory sector provision similarly implied the increasing involvement in service planning and delivery of independent sector providers.

At the same time, Griffiths set about defining more clearly the role of central as well as local government. Thus he envisaged that the centre would appoint a minister responsible for defining explicit objectives, determining priorities, publishing costed annual programmes and identifying adequate resources to fulfil those programmes through the specific grant mechanism. He argued that such a degree of control was the minimum necessary to justify the claim to have a national policy worthy of the name. What he was asserting was, in effect, the need for central government to accept its own responsibilities in this field and to exercise them through the planning process. In other words, planning was the mechanism by which he sought to ensure that the centre would both be seen to own the policy and also be seen to have its hand, however lightly, on the tiller of implementation. As we have noted, such a 'hands on' approach had not been characteristic of central government in the 1980s. Not only did this contribute to the modification of Griffiths' proposals for community care planning in the White Paper, but it has also posed continuing dilemmas about the purpose of such planning and its role in linking needs and resources.

Caring for people

After a period of some 15 months, during which alternatives to the Griffiths framework were actively sought, the government followed the broad thrust of his proposals. A number of recommendations were not accepted, however, leading Griffiths (1989) to describe the White Paper as a 'three-wheeled' version of the vehicle he had designed. Significantly, these design modifications were primarily concerned with the role of central government, including financial arrangements. Most particularly, they included the rejection of the proposals for a specific grant and for grant receipt to be conditional on the submission and approval of the community care plan. Nonetheless, and as one of the seven 'key changes' outlined in the White Paper, the 1990 NHS and Community Care Act did place local authorities under a statutory requirement to prepare, consult on and publish annual community care plans. Such plans were, however, only 'open to inspection' by the Department of Health and not to be submitted for approval by it. Three fundamental consequences flowed from these departures from the Griffiths framework: first, there would be no direct link between resource allocations from the centre and locally identified needs as expressed in community care plans; second, the responsibilities of the centre would be less transparent, since plan approval effectively represented a shared ownership of both the levels of need identified locally and also their resource implications; and third, there would be no direct financial imperative for local authorities to develop joint plans with the NHS.

This continued reliance on inter-agency coordination and collaborative planning, without any firm measure of control, was greeted with much scepticism by some commentators, who saw echoes of previous exhortations for partnership in circumstances in which partisanship was more the norm (see, for example, Hudson, 1990; Tomlinson and Nocon, 1990). The disappointing history of joint planning has been well documented elsewhere, although its apparent failings seem less marked if judged by more realistic criteria than those existing at the inception of formal joint planning in the mid-1970s (Wistow, 1988, 1990; Hardy *et al.*, 1989). Nevertheless, there would seem to have been good grounds for at least being cautious about the prospects for improved inter-agency coordination and planning in the post-White Paper context of the legislation and subsequent departmental policy guidance (see Wistow 1992, 1993). This was not just because of the previous record but also because the new context was likely to be more difficult in a number of respects. First, there was a significant increase in the number and variety of agencies involved and, second, the purchaser–provider relationship within and between agencies was untested. Moreover, the purchaser–provider framework had significant implications for the planning process itself. Indeed, the principal purpose of the purchasing role was to make more explicit decisions about planning and resource allocation. Unfortunately, however, this new framework 'required the strengthening of precisely those elements of planning which [had] been most weakly developed in the past; the analysis of needs; the specification of objectives; the setting of standards; and the evaluation of outcome' (Wistow, 1990: para. 5.5).

The scale of the demands implicit in community care planning, relative to authorities' existing planning capacities, was reflected in the Department of Health's (1990) acknowledgement that 'the development of planning would be "evolutionary" and that further advice on good practice . . . would follow' (paras 2.4 and 2.6) As we note below, such guidance has not in fact ever been published. In the event, authorities had a further twelve months to develop their planning capacities. The government's decision to phase the implementation of the 1990 Act put back the date for publishing the first plans from April 1991 to April 1992.

Community care planning: The first round

With the completion of the first round of planning, it is now possible to form some assessment of both the process and content of the plans. Such an assessment also allows judgements to be made about the purposes which the plans are and are not able to fulfil within the overall framework, contained in the White Paper, for the management and development of community care. Two principal sources of data form the basis for these assessments: first, a development programme conducted during 1991 to equip multi-agency planning teams in a number of localities to undertake their planning tasks; and, second, a detailed content analysis of a representative sample of the first plans. The first source (Wistow *et al.*, 1991) revealed that, contrary to some of the expectations outlined above, the requirement to produce plans had led to a revitalization of inter-agency planning. Thus the legislation and guidance were a catalyst to the review of joint planning arrangements which had become moribund. Building on inherited joint consultative committee planning structures, the reviews led to the tighter specification of roles, responsibilities and remits on the one hand, and the development of stronger and more explicit arrangements to secure accountability within the planning machinery on the other. Allied to this more managerialist approach to the design of planning arrangements was the development of new approaches to secure a wider range of user and carer views. However, the shift to needs-led planning was scarcely evident. Generally, localities were strong on developing agreed statements of values of principles but weak on the creation of joint information bases about needs, resources and outcomes. It was evident, therefore, that by the middle of 1991, attention had been primarily focused on the 'nuts and bolts' of planning structures and processes. Perhaps understandably, rather less attention had been given to the content of the plans.

Information on the latter is provided by our subsequent analysis of a representative sample of twenty-two English local authority plans (see Wistow *et al.*, 1993). In the first instance, the plans were analysed in terms of the four basic requirements contained in the legislation and guidance relating to publication, consultation, accessibility and 'jointness'. Beyond that, the guidance on content described a continuous process of planning and review involving the annual setting of targets and priorities through which needs and resources would be aligned (Department of Health, 1990). In respect of the initial four requirements, our findings may be summarized as follows. Each plan had been published by the 1 April 1992 deadline, a deadline not met by only one of the authorities outside the sample (Mawhinney, 1992). On consultation, we found wide variations in both the arrangements described and the detail of their description. In only a minority of cases did the consultations pre-date the preparation of the draft plans and only one of the plans gave any indication of the impact of consultations on its final form and content. Moreover, in no case was there any evidence of how satisfied those consulted had been with either the process or outcome of consultation. However, the independent sector had already made representations to the Department of Health about their dissatisfaction with consultation arrangements, following which the department commissioned from KPMG an in-depth study of independent sector involvement in planning. KPMG found that 'participative processes are widespread in terms of involving the voluntary sector but with very little involvement of private sector providers' (KPMG, 1992: para. 2.7). This finding was followed by the publication of a ministerial directive on consultation which requires authorities to consult with representatives of independent sector providers in future planning rounds (Department of Health, 1993a).

Despite the KPMG findings about voluntary sector involvement, other sources have expressed reservations about its extent. For example, Young (1992: 10) concluded that satisfaction was low 'where there were no clear "plans to plan" for the coming year and where there was very little feedback on the responses made this year'. Glendinning and Bewley's (1992) analysis of involvement by physically disabled people found that in only a minority of authorities were such arrangements well developed. However, there is good reason to be cautious about judging the effectiveness of involvement against criteria which might appear unrealistic in the first year of developing a new planning process. Whatever their limitations, the plans have been the product of more systematic consultation arrangements than have existed hitherto.

Both *Caring for People* (Department of Health, 1989) and the policy guidance (Department of Health, 1990) emphasized the importance of plans being accessible, the latter urging authorities to make them readily understandable to the public and to consider making them available in 'languages relevant to local populations' and in formats such as braille and tape (Department of Health, 1990: paras 2.18 and 2.20). Our analysis of plans found that fewer than half our sample contained summaries and only a similar proportion contained glossaries, both features which might be expected to improve the accessibility of plans. Even fewer contained sections published in languages other than English or in formats other than the written word (18 per cent in each case).

The final requirement, about the joint nature of planning, was central to the implementation of the White Paper's objectives, as the then Minister of Health emphasized in her foreword to the policy guidance (Department of Health, 1990). The guidance, itself, stressed that authorities should 'take a joint approach to planning and ensure their plans are complementary' (ibid.: para. 2.3). They should also jointly produce 'at an early stage' inventories of needs and resources, thereby allowing them to reach agreement on 'the key issues of who does what, for whom, at what cost, and who pays' (ibid.: para. 2.11). Within the sample, there was a higher proportion of joint plans: 55 per cent were jointly signed by health and local authorities; another 9 per cent were otherwise jointly agreed;

and 27 per cent showed clear evidence of complementarity with other agencies' plans. Only two plans were single agency documents.

These findings could be considered notable in view of the disappointing history of joint planning referred to above. They are consistent with the findings of an Association of Directors of Social Services report (1992) that 'the work of putting together community care plans had either cemented relationships which were already good or it had created new relationships, particularly with the FHSAs'. However, a number of caveats about our own findings are necessary. First, there was little evidence of authorities having produced detailed agreements about their respective roles and relationships. Generally, the plans simply recorded an awareness of the need to move towards clearer definitions of responsibilities and express the intention of doing so. Second, although most plans contained joint statements of values and principles, these were not always reflected in detailed objectives for individual care groups or services. Finally, it is possible that these findings, and those from our earlier development work, simply indicate that it is easier to establish planning mechanisms and secure in principle agreements about the future of cross-boundary planning than to reach agreements about funding and service responsibilities. It may, indeed, be that 1991 and 1992 will prove to be a period of 'phoney war' in advance of the transfer of social security funds (Wistow, 1994). On the other hand, the focus on broad objectives rather than specifics may also reflect the underdevelopment of the planning process as a whole, an issue to which we now turn.

While analyses of written plans alone cannot fully reveal the nature or quality of planning processes, the plans in our sample indicate authorities' progress towards the production of documents consistent with generally understood definitions of planning. Although not expressed in such terms, the policy guidance reflected a view of planning as a generic activity, the core elements of which may be described in simplified form as: determining aims and objectives; identifying and allocating resources to secure those aims and objectives; and reviewing performance and reformulating aims and objectives. (The components of this process are described more fully in Wistow, 1990: para. 5.6.) Our overall conclusion is that the first-round plans were strong on the first of those elements but weak on the other two. Their principal focus was on describing current services and identifying desired futures in broad terms, rarely indicating how such futures could be realized. Few contained costed action plans and the majority referred to resource issues only in stressing the difficulties of planning without firm resource assumptions. Moreover, few were based upon the sort of systematic analysis and alignment of needs and resources that underpinned the Griffiths Report (1988) and was reflected in the White Paper and the policy guidance. Most plans contained general service inventories – or service descriptions – rather than detailed resource inventories, from which it was clear, *inter alia*, that the mapping of independent sector supply in particular was in its infancy. Mapping of current need was similarly limited: very few authorities sought to draw upon a range of data about need and even fewer sought to predict future need. Moreover, few authorities had developed shared information systems upon which to base joint mapping of needs and resources. Our overall conclusion, therefore, was that the majority of first-round plans comprised position statements, rather than documents seeking to anticipate and change the future through the commitment of specified resources to meet identified needs.

If these seem like a catalogue of failures or shortcomings, it is important to make a number of qualifications. First, the plans were historical documents by the time our study was commissioned in September 1992 and cannot accurately reflect authorities' subsequently developed planning capacities. Second, since the plans were first prepared, there has been a large amount of central guidance, notably the two Foster/Laming letters (Department of Health, 1992a, 1992b). On the basis of the latter, it might be reasonable to surmise that authorities have, for example, moved from generalized statements of intent to more explicit definitions of authority responsibilities as a result of the requirement to sign hospital discharge and assessment agreements by 31 December 1992. It is also important to underline the low base of planning experience – and planning resources – from which most local authorities were operating. Unlike the long-established tradition of planning in the health service, national planning systems for the personal social services have, as indicated earlier, remained dormant for more than a decade – other than in the minority of authorities with medium-term corporate planning frameworks. In such circumstances, it would be inappropriate to be over-critical of limited progress in the initial planning round. However, our analysis suggests a number of priorities for future action.

Planning community care planning for the 1990s – and beyond

The first imperative in planning for community care is to recognize that the planning process itself needs to be planned as explicitly and as systematically as the development of care services. Two fundamental aspects of any planning process are that it is a continuous one, within which plans are only intermittent outputs, and that it is a prospective exercise aimed at both anticipating and shaping the future. Starting from this understanding of planning as a generic activity and applying it to our analysis of the initial plans, the following specific priorities emerge for the further development of the planning process:

• defining objectives in terms of user outcomes;
• comprehensive mapping of needs and the aggregation of population-level data with that from individual assessments;

- comprehensive mapping of supply;
- developing purchasing strategies and frameworks;
- clearly defining agency roles and responsibilities;
- integrating service and financial planning;
- monitoring and reviewing the planning process.

Addressing each of the above issues would produce a planning process which was technically equipped to produce plans rather than position statements. However, beyond such technical considerations are more fundamental questions about the intended purpose and role of planning. In turn, such questions lead us back to the very issues about the respective roles and responsibilities of central and local agencies whose necessary clarification lay at the heart of the Griffiths framework. Such issues are, moreover, inherently political not technical, as is suggested by both the delay in replying to Griffiths and also the significant departures from his recommendations to which we referred above. Similar considerations lay beneath the differences of opinion about the desirable degree of prescription in the policy guidance on planning to which Shreeve (1990) refers. They may also be assumed to have influenced the Department of Health's decision not to produce the promised (Department of Health, 1990: para. 2.6) practice guidance, an issue of some significance given the substantial volume of such guidance on every other aspect of the changes.

The same questions about the purpose and role of planning are now surfacing again in a debate about the aggregation of data from individual assessments for planning purposes. The Griffiths Report (1988) was clear that the fundamental purposes of community care plans were to serve as (1) instruments for linking needs assessment with resource allocation and (2) instruments for securing accountability. The first of these two purposes implies that authorities aggregate data about need, including unmet need, for planning in future years. Needs-led planning must, by definition, build upon both population-level and individual assessments of need.

In oral evidence to the House of Commons Health Committee (27 January 1993), the Chief Social Services Inspector emphasized the role of community care plans in drawing together such information for that purpose: 'The plan . . . is about mapping out needs within the locality . . . It is also about mapping out local resources and opportunities to meet those needs.' At the same time, however, guidance from the same source (Department of Health, 1992c) left at least some authorities concerned that they may be open to legal challenge if they record unmet individual needs. As one director of social services remarked: 'I can well understand there may be judicial reviews coming out of all this. I don't want local authorities to be liable simply because of information placed on a form' (Cohen, 1993). Nor was this concern lessened by a subsequent letter from the Social Services Inspectorate (Department of Health, 1993b) suggesting the recording of unmet choice rather than unmet need, a distinction described by one director of social services as 'bizarre' (Watt, 1993).

Moreover, the Department of Health has indicated that it will not be collecting and collating information about unmet need from the community care plans. The Association of Directors of Social Services, however, has suggested that, in those circumstances, such data 'will be added up for them [the Department]' (Neate, 1993). In a House of Commons debate, one of the government's own backbenchers, Roger Sims, spoke of his anxiety about unmet need being unrecorded; a concern based upon evidence to the Health Committee by Department of Health officials. This, he said, 'negates the whole principle that community care should be driven by needs rather than resources' (House of Commons, 1993). He asked how the department could know that resources were adequate 'without having information about unmet need'. Acknowledging that funds were not unlimited, he argued that:

> ... we should all know where we stand. The local authority should have it on record and know the exact position. It should know not only the needs that it is meeting, but the needs that it has been unable to meet. Those statistics could then be collected at Richmond House and my right hon. and hon. Friends the Ministers will be able to see whether community care is working.
>
> (House of Commons, 1993)

It is self-evident that no government could be expected to meet all needs. Equally, however, it is difficult to understand how planning and resource allocation can be needs-led unless such information is systematically sought out, explicitly recorded and fed into planning processes at central as well as local government level. It is at this point that Griffiths' second basic purpose of planning – that of accountability – becomes relevant. As noted above, Griffiths argued that he was proposing a minimum degree of control consistent with there being a national policy worthy of that name. It is perhaps significant, if not ironic, that in developing a coherent national implementation strategy for the community care changes, the Department of Health effectively reinvented parts of Griffiths: a limited form of ringfencing was introduced and payment of the transfer resources so transferred was conditional upon local and health authorities submitting signed agreements on arrangements for hospital discharges and the purchase of nursing home care. It is hard to escape the conclusion that something approaching the Griffiths framework is necessary if a shared ownership of the implementation of the community care changes is to be continued. If central government is not to collect information about need, that partnership – and more fundamentally the Department of Health's commitment to the needs-led development of services – must equally be under question. Griffiths himself lamented the fact that community care was 'everybody's poor relation and nobody's baby' (Griffiths, 1988). The role of community care plans in making more explicit the relationship between needs and resources is a major test case of the extent to which central and local agencies accept their separate and joint responsibilities for parenthood.

References

Association of Directors of Social Services (1992). *Maintaining Change in Social Services Departments.* London: ADSS.

Audit Commission (1986). *Making a Reality of Community Care.* London: HMSO.

Cohen, P. (1993). Directors seek legal advice on assessments. *Social Work Today,* 4 February, p. 3.

Department of Health (1989). *Caring for People: Community Care in the Next Decade and Beyond.* Cm. 849. London: HMSO.

Department of Health (1990). *Community Care in the Next Decade and Beyond: Policy Guidance.* London: HMSO.

Department of Health (1992a). *Implementing Caring for People.* EL(92)13/Cl(92)10; 11 March.

Department of Health (1992b). *Implementing Caring for People.* EL(92)65/Cl(92)30; 25 September.

Department of Health (1992c). *Implementing Caring for People: Assessment.* Cl(92)34.

Department of Health (1993a). *Community Care Plans (Consultation) Directions 1993,* 25 January 1993. London: Department of Health.

Department of Health (1993b). *Implementing Caring for People: Assessment.* Letter to London Directors of Social Services, 1 March.

Department of Health and Social Security (1972). *Local Authority Social Services Ten Year Development Plans 1973–1983.* Circular 35/72. London: DHSS.

Department of Health and Social Security (1976). *Priorities for Health and Personal Social Services in England: A Consultative Document.* London: HMSO.

Glendinning, C. and Bewley, C. (1992). *Involving Disabled People in Community Care Planning – The First Steps: An Analysis of Community Care Plans for England and Wales 1992.* Manchester: Department of Social Policy and Social Work, University of Manchester.

Griffiths, R. (1988). *Community Care: Agenda for Action.* London: HMSO.

Griffiths, R. (1989). Speech to National Association of Health Authorities. London: HMSO.

Hardy, B., Turrell, A., Webb, A. and Wistow, G. (1989). *Collaboration and Cost Effectiveness: Final Report.* Loughborough: Centre for Research in Social Policy, Loughborough University.

House of Commons (1993). *Proceedings,* 11 February, Columns 1145–1146.

House of Commons Social Services Committee (1985). *Community Care with Special Reference to Adult Mentally Ill and Mentally Handicapped People.* HC 13 Session 1984–85. London: HMSO.

Hudson, B. (1990). Yes, but will it work? *The Health Service Journal,* 1 February, pp. 169–70.

KPMG (1992). *Improving Independent Sector Involvement in Community Care Planning.* A Report for the Department of Health. London: Department of Health.

Mawhinney, B. (1992). Speech by Minister of Health to the IHSM/ADSS Conference, London, 10 July, para. 8. London: Department of Health.

Ministry of Health (1962). *A Hospital Plan for England and Wales.* Cmnd 1604. London: HMSO.

Ministry of Health (1963). *The Development of Community Care.* Cmnd 1973. London: HMSO.

National Audit Office (1987). *Community Care Developments.* London: HMSO.

Neate, P. (1993). Time to bed down the reforms. *Community Care,* 4 March, p. 10.

Shreeve, M. (1990). Community care planning and mental illness specific grant: Issues in the draft circulars. In Allen, I. (ed.), *Community Care Planning and Mental Illness Specific Grant.* London: PSI.

Tomlinson, D. and Nocon, A. (1990). The day of reckoning draws nigh. *Health Services Management,* August, pp. 189–91.

Watt, S. (1993). Directors stunned over unmet needs. *Care Weekly,* 11 March, p. 1.

Webb, A. and Wistow, G. (1982). *Whither State Welfare? Policy and Implementation in the Personal Social Services 1979–80.* London: Royal Institute of Public Administration.

Webb, A. and Wistow, G. (1986). *Planning, Need and Scarcity: Essays on the Personal Social Services.* London: Allen and Unwin.

Wistow, G. (1988). Health and local authority collaboration: Lessons and prospects. In Wistow, G. and Brookes, T. (eds), *Joint Planning and Joint Management.* London: Royal Institute of Public Administration.

Wistow, G. (1990). *Community Care Planning: A Review of Past Experience and Future Imperatives.* Caring for People Implementation Document CC13. London: Department of Health.

Wistow, G. (1992). Working together in a new policy context. *Health Services Management,* February, pp. 25–8.

Wistow, G. (1993). *Working Together After the Health and Social Care Reforms.* Second Smith and Nephew Foundation Lecture, University of Hull: Department of Social Policy and Professional Studies.

Wistow, G. (1994). Community Care Futures. Inter-agency relationships: Stability or continuing change? In Titterton, M. (ed.), *Caring for People in the Community: The New Welfare.* London: Jessica Kingsley.

Wistow, G. and Henwood, M. (1989). Planning in a mixed economy. In Parry, R. (ed.), *Privatisation.* London: Jessica Kingsley.

Wistow, G., Swift, J. and Hallas, J. (1991). Community care planning workshops: *Caring for People, 8,* 14, 16.

Wistow, G., Leedham, I. and Hardy, B. (1993). *Implementing Community Care: Community Care Plans.* London: Department of Health, Social Services Inspectorate.

Young, C. (1992). Community care plans in the shire counties. In *The First Plans: Some Views of the Initial Community Care Planning Process,* p. 10. London: NCVO.

4 Care management

David Challis

Introduction

Major developments in long-term care are occurring in many countries and some broadly similar trends can be discerned. In their study of emerging patterns of change in services for elderly people in the Netherlands, Sweden and the UK, Kraan *et al.* (1991) noted a move away from institution-based care, the enhancement of home-based care and the development of mechanisms of coordination and case management. In the care of elderly people in many other countries such as the USA, Canada and Australia, a similar trend can also be observed (Challis, 1992a, 1992b). In the mental health services, the reduction of institutional provision and focus upon community-based services is clear (Huxley *et al.*, 1990). Long-term care policy for other client groups has also taken not dissimilar forms, with the desire to develop community services being stressed (Department of Health, 1989; DHSS, 1983). Underlying this is a major debate about the extent to which community services complement or are a substitute for institutional care.

Concern for coordination has been longstanding and in the UK took the form principally of attempts to improve inter-agency coordination, principally health and social care, through such initiatives as joint care planning and joint financing. The focus upon coordination at the client level came considerably later, being less evident in a setting where most services were provided by two main agencies, health and social services. For people with a mental handicap or a learning disability in the USA, discharge from hospital and developing continuity of care have been key themes, with case management made mandatory to improve coordination of care after discharge (Intagliata, 1982). The rationale for this is cited by Miller (1983), who quotes the conclusion of the US Presidential Commission on Mental Health for case management: 'Strategies focused solely on organisations are not enough. A human link is required. A case manager can provide this link and assist in assuring continuity of care and a coordinated program of services' (pp. 5–6).

In general, therefore, the origins of case management lie in the 'need to coordinate delivery of long-term care services to individual clients' (Austin, 1983). Moxley (1989) cites six factors underlying the development of case management: deinstitutionalization; the decentralized nature of community services; growing numbers of clients with multiple needs living at home; the fragmentation of care services; a growing awareness of the importance of social supports and carers; and the need for cost containment. Case management and coordination are thus central to the achievement of the goals of community-based care.

Case management is thus in a crucial position in the new care arrangements, being the mechanism designed to achieve both the move away from institutional provision and the strengthening of home-based care. It is the point at which welfare objectives and resource constraints are closest together. Therefore, case management has a pivotal role as the setting where the integration of social and economic criteria must occur at the level of service provision, where the balancing of needs and resources, scarcity and choice must take place (Challis, 1992b). It should not be seen as a panacea (Callahan, 1989) nor a 'silver bullet' (Austin, 1992) for the ills of community care, but rather a particular device which, dependent upon the manner of its implementation, offers a means to manage some intractable policy and practice dilemmas.

Hence a great deal is dependent upon the coherence, form, style and structure of the case management processes implemented to effect community care changes in many countries. This chapter attempts to clarify and define the nature of case management and to consider some factors that appear to be associated with more or less effective implementation.

Case or care management

The definition of case management is far from easy. Definitions abound and even terminology changes. Thus the Griffiths Report (1988) talked of 'care management', and the subsequent White Paper (Department of Health, 1989) used the term 'case management'. Later, the Department of Health (1991a, 1991b) guidelines published for managers and practitioners refer to 'care' management, justifying this in terms of the fact that it is the care which is being managed and that the word case may be perceived as demeaning. A similar point is made in the Care Management Standards of the National Institute on Community-Based Long-Term Care (1988) in the USA. The debate about nomenclature occurs elsewhere too. One major organization in the USA, Connecticut Community Care, uses the words 'care management' and 'care managers'; alternatively, the State of Wisconsin provides a 'care management program' but employs the terms 'care manager' and 'case manager' interchangeably, whereas Washington State uses the term 'case management'. Conversely, in the Canadian Province of Manitoba, the term 'case coordinator' is employed (Fineman, 1992), and recently in British Columbia the term 'assessor' in the continuing care programme has been changed to 'case manager', reflecting increasing dependency in the needs of the primary client population and the need for continuity of care (British Columbia Ministry of Health, 1992). What is important is less the precise terms which are used and more the clarity of meaning which is attached to different aspects of the process. Here, the terms will be used interchangeably, although 'care management' as a general process and 'case management' as a client level activity might be preferable.

The origins of case management, then, lie in the immediate need for coordination of home-based care, albeit with a broader range of objectives including client-centred care and effective use of resources (Challis, 1992b). How may case management be best defined? Definitions of case management usually revolve around a statement of functions, specification of core tasks, goals which it is designed to achieve, key differentiating features, delineation of the recipients of the service and identification of the context within which it takes place. Each of these would seem to be an important component of its definition.

Functions of case management

In overall functional terms, Austin (1983: 16) defines case management as '. . . a mechanism for linking and coordinating segments of a service delivery system . . . to ensure the most comprehensive programme for meeting an individual's needs for care'. This involves continuity of involvement and is based upon comprehensive assessment of the individual's needs (Kane, 1990). Moxley (1989: 17) usefully defines case management as '. . . a dedicated person (or team) who organises, coordinates and sustains a network of formal and informal supports and activities designed to optimise the functioning and well-being of people with multiple needs'. More generally, Modricin *et al.* (1988: 307) describe it as the achievement of a better fit between '. . . the person's needs and the resources available in the community'. The Department of Health (1991a: 11) guidance defines care management as '. . . the process of tailoring services to individual needs'. It then refers to specific care tasks.

Specified core tasks

A second common feature of the definition of case management involves the performance of a series of core tasks in long-term care (Steinberg and

Carter, 1983; Department of Health, 1991a, 1991b). There is some variation in the precise description of these, for example the Department of
Health has included 'publishing information', which elsewhere might be
considered as part of case-finding. The Province of British Columbia defines case management as '. . . a specific set of client-related functions that
include intake and screening for eligibility, assessment of functions and
needs, mutual service planning and goal setting, efficient linkage with
available resources, quality assurance through ongoing monitoring, review
and evaluation, and discharge policy' (British Columbia Ministry of Health,
1992). Overall, there would seem to be across the literature a broad general
consensus. These core tasks are case finding and screening, assessment,
care planning, implementing and monitoring the care plan. As such, these
core tasks may usefully be differentiated from more short-term activities of
care providers (Challis *et al.*, 1990). However, case management is more
than a set of processes in long term-care, since in undertaking these tasks
also involves advocacy and integrating formal and informal care (Capitman
et al., 1986).

Goals of case management

These most usually involve specifying coordination of community-based
services, sometimes without reference to the importance of its role at the
margin between modes of care, institutional and home-based care, reflecting the varied target populations of case management services. Moxley
(1989) notes three goals of case management: improving client utilization
of support and services; developing the capacity of social networks and
services to promote client well-being; and promoting service effectiveness
and efficiency. These are similar to those cited by the National Institute
for Community-Based Long-Term Care (1988) in the USA, which cover
both client-centred activities such as enhanced service access, coordinated care, independence and community tenure, as well as more system-
focused goals such as improved service availability, reaching a specified
target population and cost containment through the use of appropriate
community-based services. These recognize the potential for goal conflict
such as between client and carer or between cost containment and client
responsiveness, and specify the need for mechanisms to resolve such conflicts. These include family meetings, advocacy, case manager peer group
support and effective supervision.

Thus the objectives of case management can be seen as very similar to
those identified for community mental health services in the USA and the
UK: comprehensiveness, coordination, access, acceptability, efficiency,
effectiveness and accountability (Huxley *et al.*, 1990).

Key differentiating features of case management

Applebaum and Austin (1990) note that many organizations report that they do case management and that they do undertake some of the relevant activities. In the US context, it has been argued that case management is what most social workers do in most fields of practice most of the time (Roberts-DeGennaro, 1987). In the UK, an obvious example of this is the role of the key worker within multidisciplinary teams. However, there are important differences between these key worker approaches, which aim to coordinate a *single service or team* more appropriately to individual needs, often on a short-term basis, and case management, which aims to coordinate *multiple services and providers*, usually on a *long-term* basis. Applebaum and Austin (1990) identify three factors which differentiate long-term care case management from these key worker approaches. These are intensity of involvement, reflected in relatively small caseloads; breadth of services spanned, covering more than one service, team or agency; and length or duration of involvement, being a long-term commitment. In the *Care Management Standards* documentation of the National Institute of Community-Based Long-Term Care (1988), a similar distinction is made between single agency coordination and comprehensive case management, which is '. . . an inclusive look across a person's needs and resources, linking him or her to a full range of appropriate services, using all available funding sources and monitoring the care provided over an extended period of time'.

Recipients of case management services

Another key element is that case management is concerned with meeting the needs of people with long-term care problems or multiple needs (Steinberg and Carter, 1983; Moxley, 1989). The definition of this group is not easy. Davies and Challis (1986) characterize long-term care populations as: those using a high proportion of health and social care expenditure; individuals with multiple and varied needs; recipients of multiple and inflexible services of which social care is the largest component. Ballew and Mink (1986) describe case management as concerned with people experiencing multiple problems that require multiple sources of help, and who experience difficulty in utilizing that help. The role of case management is thus seen as combining brokerage with interpersonal skills, since it is focused both '. . . on the network of services needed by multi-problem clients and the interaction between members of the network' (ibid.: p. 8). Therefore, case management is concerned with providing services to a specific target group and need not be seen as the mechanism for providing all forms of care for those who need assistance in coping with everyday living (Kane, 1990). This specificity is evident in the application of case management to community care developments in a number of countries (Challis, 1992a, 1992b).

Organizational context of case management

Thus, the definition includes comprehensive assessment, continuity, coordination, the performance of the core tasks of case management and the meeting of needs for a long-term care population, hence providing services to a specific target group. A final but crucial contextual element is identified by Miller (1983), who notes that a focus on client-level activities is insufficient, since it does not address the idea of a case management system. Similarly, O'Connor (1988) makes the distinction between case management practice and case management systems. As Moore (1990) argues, the degree of horizontal integration achieved by case management practice needs a degree of vertical integration at the system level in order to be effective. Kane (1990) links case management practice with system-level activities through the use of comprehensive assessments to provide aggregated information for needs-based planning by agencies. In short, case management is designed not just to influence care at the individual client level, but also at the system level through the aggregate of a myriad of care decisions at the individual client level which exert pressure for change upon patterns of provision themselves. An underlying objective is to render those patterns of services more relevant to individual needs (Austin, 1983; Steinberg and Carter, 1983; Department of Health, 1991b).

Let us now examine some of the experience of case management developments for some indicators of effective implementation.

Common problems of implementation

There are clearly shared concerns expressed regarding the implementation of case management. Table 1 summarizes those concerns identified in most of the available UK work and some studies from overseas. The latter three are selected because of their more general importance. The Wisconsin Mental Health Programme has been implemented in several other parts of the USA and elsewhere (Hoult *et al.*, 1983; Stein and Test, 1985; Hoult, 1990), the Wisconsin Community Options Programme (McDowell *et al.*, 1990) has been very influential in the development of case management in Australia and the Channelling Programme was a major US national demonstration study (Kemper, 1988; Weissert, 1988).

Implementation problems in case management

In the implementation of community care, the Audit Commission (1992a) have indicated several progressive stages to be accomplished, but observe

Table 1 Implementation concerns in care management from different studies

	1	2	3	4	5	6	7	8	9	10
Targeting	×	×	×	×	–	–	×	×	×	×
Caseload size	×	×	×	–	–	–	–	×	×	×
Location of case management	×	×	×	×	×	–	–	×	–	–
Brokerage or more extensive approaches	×	×	×	×	–	×	–	×	×	×
Influence upon service providers	×	×	×	×	–	×	×	×	×	×
Management, standards and quality assurance	×	×	×	×	×	–	×	–	×	–
Logical coherence of case management arrangements	×	×	×	–	×	–	–	×	×	–

KEY
1. Thanet community care scheme (Challis and Davies, 1986; Davies and Challis, 1986)
2. Gateshead community care scheme (Challis *et al.*, 1988, 1990, 1992)
3. Darlington community care project (Challis *et al.*, 1989, 1991a, 1991b)
4. Gloucester care of elderly people at home project (Dant *et al.*, 1989)
5. Wakefield case management scheme (Richardson and Higgins, 1990, 1992)
6. Choice case management service (Pilling, 1988, 1992)
7. Andover case management project (National Development Team, 1991)
8. Wisconsin PACT mental health service (Stein and Test, 1980, 1985; Test and Stein, 1980; Weisbrod *et al.*, 1980; Stein, Diamond and Factor, 1989)
9. Wisconsin community options programme (McDowell *et al.*, 1990)
10. Review of US Channelling Programme for the elderly (Kemper, 1988; Weissert, 1988)

that care management poses the greatest challenge describing it as the 'lynchpin of the new system of community care' (p. 33). They list a range of decisions to be taken, including the scope of care management (who will receive it), the size of caseloads and numbers of case managers required, their degree of influence over services, the degree of budget devolution, whether case managers should function as specialist or generic workers, and the financial and management information required by care managers. These concerns correspond to a considerable extent with those major issues identified from earlier work in Fig. 1. Let us now examine these in more detail.

Targeting

Defining which people are appropriate for care management is a major theme, since not all users of care services will require or permit the overhead cost of a case manager. In the UK, this requires us to make a distinction between 'intensive case management' for a limited group and a 'care management approach' across the service system. This distinction is fundamental and commences with targeting. Two different aspects of targeting have been discussed – case-finding and screening (Challis and Davies, 1986; Davies and Challis, 1986). Austin (1981) has referred to these as effective and efficient targeting. Screening is crucial to policies for achieving a degree of substitution of institutional care by home care. Thus some of the success of the Thanet, Gateshead and Darlington (Challis and Davies, 1985, 1986; Challis *et al.*, 1988, 1989, 1991a, 1991b, 1993) case management services for elderly people must be attributed to their having been appropriately targeted, focused upon people with considerable needs and a high probability of entry to institutional care. Indeed, much of the difficulty of case management demonstrations has been to achieve the degree of desired downward substitution, as well as showing welfare gains among those receiving the service, has been attributed to problems of targeting (Kemper, 1988; Hennessy and Hennessy, 1990). Similarly, in reviewing 14 US case management programmes for the chronically mentally ill, Huxley (1991) has noted that a narrow and specific target group definition is associated with reduced institutional care and positive outcomes. The consequences of not targeting intensive care management on the most needy could, in the context of the UK community care changes, lead to the paradox of an unplanned continuing switch of resources from domiciliary services to residential and nursing home care.

However, the implementation of acceptable procedures for ensuring eligibility is complex. It will be important to ensure that those who receive case management are those for whom the service is designed. The apparent equity and ease of implementation of methods such as relatively simple screening schedules have to be balanced against considerations of reliability and validity. A focus of concern is with individuals liable to enter institutional care and factors that make coping in the community problematic. In practice, this has meant balancing objective and apparently equitable criteria with a degree of discretion which reflects the complexity of life situations. The Audit Commission (1992a) cite four target populations as suitable for care management: those at high risk of entry to institutional care (including those with chronic mental health problems); those with stressed informal carers; those requiring resettlement from long-stay institutions; and those requiring intensive short-term support following illness or injury. A review of twenty long-term care management projects noted that the most common client-related eligibility criteria were: functional impairment ($n = 14$), risk of nursing home placement ($n = 10$), potential for nursing home discharge ($n = 8$) and hospital discharge ($n = 7$) (Applebaum and Austin, 1990). In the Wisconsin Community Options Case Management Programme, the same criteria are used both to assess eligibility for the case management programme as for nursing homes (McDowell *et al.*, 1990). These criteria include the presence of a severe unstable medical condition and long-term illness, or substantial medical and social needs including the inability to perform activities of daily living, or a need for supervision and care, usually for people with dementia (Community Options Programme, 1992). The attraction of such a system is that where case management is seen as providing an alternative option of home care to nursing home care, it is clear that equivalent criteria are being employed and this process was associated with one of the most effectively targeted case management services in the US channelling demonstration (Applebaum and Austin, 1990). Other US states with broader eligibility criteria use a range of activities of daily living indicators (Luehrs and Ramthun, 1991); however, even well-validated indicators tend to be quite variable when used in non-experimental and less controlled practice environments (Liu and Cornelius, 1991). This is particularly problematic since apparently objective indicators of dependency are insufficient as predictors of the probability of entry to residential or nursing home care (Neill *et al.*, 1988; Luehrs and Ramthun, 1991). Indeed, Applebaum and Austin (1990) observe that for every individual with certain ADL score entering nursing home care, there were two with similar levels of disability remaining at home. Kane (1988a) has noted the danger of further tightening entry criteria to only accept those who said they were applicants for nursing home entry, since the administration of such an approach would render worthless any predictive value that such an application might have had.

The lack of reliable, valid and efficient indicators of need for institutional care suggests the combination of a general eligibility criterion of need for services with the exercise of discretion over which service mode any given individual receives. In the Wisconsin Mental Health Programme (Stein and Test, 1985), where the target population was individuals with chronic mental health problems, neither diagnosis nor severity of illness were seen as sufficient indicators, although most patients suffered from schizophrenia. Rather, the focus was upon the specific determinants of service mix. Seven criteria were identified: willingness to come for services; compliance with medication; need for structured daily activities; ability to self-monitor; frequency of crises; need for professional psychological support; and degree of case management (Stein *et al.*, 1989). In some Canadian provinces, several categories of need have been developed, corresponding to intensity of service provision, but allocation between categories involves the exercise of professional judgement rather than the use of rigid formulae (Kane and Kane, 1991). Thus in the Manitoba Home Care Programme (Fineman, 1992), three criteria determine eligibility: hospital discharge, risk of entry to hospital care or nursing home care. Similarly in the UK, some case management schemes used agreed guidelines for referral but, recognizing the complexity of circumstances which constitute conditions such as need for institutional care, no rigid pre-entry threshold of dependency was specified and accountability for targeting was monitored post-entry. Clearly, such an approach has the advantage of permitting discretion but requires careful monitoring and is potentially subject to dispute. Managerial scrutiny of such decision-making processes is necessary and requires the development of improved information systems, including information on client characteristics. The development of mechanisms for achieving effective targeting is thus likely to be linked with debates about assessment.

In the UK, there is an explicit separation of assessment and case management as the cornerstone of the new policy (Department of Health, 1989). This reflects the concern with issues of eligibility and appropriate placement of vulnerable individuals, as well as with the more effective coordination of community-based care (Department of Health, 1989, 1990). The practice and managerial guidance makes specific reference to differentiated levels of assessment and the need to determine the appropriate level of assessment for a given individual (Department of Health, 1991a, 1991b). However, although a range of possible trigger indicators (which are in effect screening tools) are discussed (Department of Health, 1991b) and some useful work has been undertaken (Lutz, 1989), there is relatively little systematic focus upon methods of pre-assessment screening to compare with the investment in assessment formats. Hence assessment as a problem identification process and screening as an eligibility judgement are discussed together as if one phenomenon, which may at times lead to a degree of confusion.

Caseload size

Targeting policy will also affect caseload size, which is likely to influence both the quality and style of case management. Indeed, this indicator is one quality standard that has been used to ensure that sufficient staff time is allocated to each case. A number of factors appear to have influenced decisions about caseload size: the characteristics of the client group served; complexity of care plans; type of area served (urban *vs* rural); degree of clerical support; availability of community services; and responsibility and control over funds (National Institute on Community-Based Long-Term Care, 1988). The caseload size in the Thanet, Gateshead and Darlington studies was around 25–30 cases; in some mental health programmes it is much lower, reflecting expectations of much greater work in human relationships such as engagement. Washington State (1986) has a maximum of 50 cases per worker in its age care programme and the average in the Wisconsin Community Options Programme is 40.

Applebaum and Austin (1990) note the variability in caseload size in the long-term care of elderly people, ranging from 35 to 85 cases per worker. They cite surveys of case managers indicating preferred caseload sizes of 30–50 cases and note the evidence of a decreasing capacity to perform follow-up, monitoring and review as caseload size increases. Clearly, there is a trade-off between caseload size and effective performance of these activities which will concern those implementing programmes in the UK. Caseload size is likely to determine the feasible style of case management (Bachrach, 1992), which is discussed later. Caseload size is, of course, more problematic to define when a team approach to case management is adopted for some particularly demanding clients in some mental health programmes (Stein *et al.*, 1989). Some US states have begun to develop caseload weighting approaches as part of their quality assurance programmes, which take into account factors such as workload, level of administrative support and type of area.

The location of care management

Case management has been located in a variety of different settings, including social services departments, hospitals, geriatric and psychiatric multidisciplinary teams, primary care, independent agencies and even independent actors. The effective implementation of case management will need to identify appropriate settings to provide case management for individuals with different kinds of needs. An examination of the extent to which different locations may or may not facilitate the performance of the core tasks can be helpful in analysing their relative advantages as settings for case management. The role of general practitioners (GPs) in screening elderly people over the age of seventy-five may identify unmet social care needs, perhaps providing case finding in a more universally acceptable setting (Challis *et al.*, 1990, 1992). Primary care may thus offer improved accessibility to the primary health care team and home support, but on the other hand the numbers of people on any one GP's list requiring case management will be small and intensive case management might be better located in secondary health care settings such as geriatric services (Challis *et al.*, 1991a, 1991b). Similarly, care for those suffering from chronic schizophrenia may be better provided as part of the community mental health service, where case managers are part of a psychiatric service. Similar arguments apply to community mental handicap teams (Audit Commission, 1992a). There may also be a case for arguing that people whose needs are relatively rare within the catchment area of one local authority may have their needs better met by a service perhaps located in a non-profit agency covering several local authorities.

In the care of elderly people, one critical factor is likely to be hospital discharge and the lack of incentives to effectively pursue this. Joint budgets and agreements are seen as a potential solution (Audit Commission, 1992a). The mid-term review of the Australian community care reforms for older people suggests the need to link care management and long-term care services to hospital discharge to prevent the risk of bed-blocking (Gregory, 1991), which suggests some advantages of health care locations.

Brokerage or more extensive models of care management

The implementation of care management sometimes appears to consider the core tasks rather more as administrative activities, involving mainly brokerage and service allocation, than integrating these with tasks such as support and counselling, which require staff with human relations skills. This is evident in discussions about the separation of purchaser and provider roles, where a rigid distinction considers the provision of human relations skills and emotional support as only a 'provider' role, although this is quite inappropriate in good practice. An alternative formulation is that of 'clinical' case management (Harris and Bergman, 1987; Kanter, 1987, 1989; Harris and Bachrach, 1988), which offers a broader combination of roles, and it seems that most services fall somewhere between these poles (Bachrach, 1992).

Studies have consistently indicated that more than brokerage functions are required in practice, even if this were not made explicit in the initial planning or job descriptions (Dant *et al.*, 1989; Applebaum and Austin, 1990; Dant and Gearing, 1990), and that case managers are successful in performing the core tasks through combining practical care with the use of human relations skills, including counselling and support, not only to carers and users but also to direct care staff (Challis and Davies, 1986; Challis *et al.*, 1988, 1989, 1990, 1991a, 1991b, 1992). Rothman (1991: 523) notes that case management '. . . incorporates two central functions: 1) Providing individualised advice, counselling and therapy to clients in the community and 2) Linking clients to needed services and supports in community agencies and informal helping networks'. In reviewing case management studies in the mental health field, Chamberlain and Rapp (1991: 185) note: 'Simplistic notions of case management as a mere brokering of service seems to have been abandoned . . . [most] studies are based on case management interventions which emphasise relationship, intensity of involvement, outreach mode of service delivery etc which were not usually included in earlier descriptions of case management'. Similarly, the British Columbia case management guide states: 'Case Managers do both direct services and allocate contracted services on behalf of clients. The direct services are generally counselling, teaching, supporting and crisis intervention' (British Columbia Ministry of Health, 1992: 25).

The US National Standards documents indicate that case managers are expected to assume most or all of the roles of service coordinator, advocate, counsellor and gatekeeper (National Institute of Community-Based Long-Term Care, 1988). Moxley (1989: 144) notes that '. . . ignoring the clinical and interpersonal practice dimensions of case management is counterproductive'. He argues that effective case management needs a caring and individualized relationship between client and case manager, the use of interpersonal skills, intervention in crises and knowledge of the clinical expertise of other disciplines. In their review of case management programmes for frail elderly people, Steinberg and Carter (1983: 139) conclude that 'Case Managers must be clinically oriented, be skilled in establishing and sustaining personal relationships, like and respect older people, be able to coordinate medical, social and instrumental needs and services, participate in assessment and carry through with implementation'.

Although there is considerable debate about the roles required of case managers and the specific skills and training which they require, it would seem that there is a scarcity of appropriately trained personnel. However, without deliberate planning such a scarcity of appropriate staff could well influence the style of case management that develops, and an explicit commitment to a clinical model of case management could act as a helpful counter to the risk of overformalization and insensitivity in the new care arrangements. This is perhaps more likely in some client groups than others. For example, it may be that a pure brokerage model is less readily accepted for people with mental health problems than it is for elderly people because of the sheer visibility of factors such as relationship difficulties.

Influence upon service providers

Crucial to the effective implementation of care management is the degree of influence which case managers have over the form and content of services provided. Arnold (1987) has argued that a brokerage model alone is insufficient to effect influence and Austin (1992: 11) criticizing pure brokerage, concludes that 'Case Managers who cannot deliver the services they prescribe in their care plans are not very likely to be very effective'. Dant and Gearing (1990) observe that effective case management requires the case manager to control the supply or availability of services and other resources, and a common conclusion is that case management should be separated from the immediate activity of service provision, to render it more client-centred than service-focused.

The separation of purchaser and provider is seen as an important part of the development of services in the UK, with case management seen as a purchaser role (Department of Health, 1990). As such, its role is designed to influence the pattern of provision in more appropriate ways. The distinction between purchaser and provider is deceptively simple and different levels of separation may be discerned. On the one hand, there is macro-purchasing, the form of purchasing most commonly associated until the present time with health authorities contracting with particular providers to provide services for a district or an area. Similarly, such purchasing procedures may be developed by local authorities, indeed, case management itself could be purchased on such a basis for particular client groups or for particular areas of the local authority. This process of managing an overall market and purchasing supply to meet the needs of a population within an area should be distinguished from the micro-purchasing role, whereby case managers individually dispense their budgets (Department of Health, 1991a). It appears that some of the most appropriate responses to needs have been made by the individualized and often idiosyncratic purchases made by case managers on behalf of their clients due to their control over resources.

There is, however, significant variation in the degree of influence over resource allocation. This has ranged from pure advocacy and negotiation (Pilling, 1988, 1992) through small 'top-up' budgets (Dant et al., 1989) to more substantial budgets close to the full revenue cost of community care (Challis and Davies, 1985, 1986; Challis et al., 1988, 1989, 1991a, 1991b, 1992). The Madison Mental Health Scheme stressed most radically the concentration of all funding (Stein, 1989; Stein et al., 1989). However, budgetary devolution can raise some difficult questions. Premature devolution of previously centralized budgets without reference to past patterns of expenditure and estimates of need is risky and the alignment of finance and management responsibility at the same level seem to be crucial (Audit Commission, 1992a). Indeed, in the State of Wisconsin, it appears that devolution of budgets was necessary as a means of effective budgetary scrutiny and control, which paradoxically was not feasible with centralized allocation and control.

However, the separation of purchaser and provider roles at the micro-level raises more problems than at the macro-level and there are dangers in the pursuit of too rigid a separation. Some roles and activities may span the purchaser/provider divide and blur an apparently clear distinction. An obvious example is that of counselling and support. Conceptually, it might be possible to define supportive counselling as a provider function, but in most settings this process – engaging a person, forming a relationship with them and comprehending the depth of their problems so as to establish the right mix of support and services which they need – proves to be a purchaser function. Indeed, to make such an activity an exclusive provider function would inevitably push care management towards an administrative or brokerage role. Thus the needs of effective practice do not always lead to organizationally neat solutions. Again in the care of a cognitively impaired elderly person, a hands-on carer (provider) might be used to contribute to assessment and other core tasks such as monitoring well-being, routine, diet or medication intake because of their proximity to the elderly person over a considerable period of time, albeit closely supported by a case manager. The complexity regarding what is defined as a service (and therefore a 'provider role') is discussed by the Department of Health (1991a), and as a consequence some schemes have attempted to define limits to activities such as counselling to limit involvement (Pilling, 1988, 1992). The nature of these relationships between provider and purchaser therefore need to be explored carefully so that the process of separation does not lead to new problems of inappropriate care. One helpful way of viewing the separation is to be clear about the different roles of case management and service management, sometimes problematically blurred in agencies, which underpin the functions of purchaser and provider at the micro level.

Management: Standards and quality

Much discussion of care management focuses upon the performance of the core tasks of case management in client-level work and upon styles and types of fieldwork practice. However, there are important issues for the management of care management, acknowledged in the separate guidance for practitioners and managers (Department of Health, 1991a, 1991b). Changes will be required in financial and monitoring systems (Audit Commission, 1992a, 1992b; Financial Management Partnership, 1992) and in the ways in which such information is deployed. Considerable effort is being devoted to system development and consolidation will take a relatively long time. Of less visibility in debates and taken up at a later stage in their development by many case management services overseas is the nature of quality assurance. In a context of greater devolution of authority and possibly flatter organizational hierarchies, there will be a need for mangers to focus less upon traditional methods of procedural adherence and more upon outcome-focused approaches; a focus more upon ends and less upon means. The focus is likely to be increasingly upon inter-agency activities as well as those at the client/worker and agency levels (Steinberg and Carter, 1983). Furthermore, the importance of managerial commitment and involvement was noted in several of the studies in Fig. 1 and has been seen to be critical in the subsequent dissemination of successful models of service (Hoult, 1990).

Consequently, at the managerial level, there will need to be a development of approaches to quality assurance and supervision which differ from much previous practice. The Department of Health (1991a) guidance for managers states that: 'Middle managers . . . will also have to develop new skills in the promotion of a more entrepreneurial approach by practitioners . . . important though cost consciousness will be it should be balanced by an appropriate concern for the quality of care that is being provided'. Where the focus of managers is only upon costs, the most easily measured and recorded indicator, perverse incentives could easily emerge, such as the manipulation of the target group by individual case managers to attract less costly cases onto their caseloads. The Department of Health's guidance argues that standards should be incorporated into the specifications for all services and such careful monitoring should also be applied to the case management process itself, as well as to the services organized by case managers. This will require the development of record systems to monitor process, cost and outcomes.

Indicators of quality have traditionally been seen as indicators of structure, process and outcome (Donabedian, 1980). *Structural* indicators are concerned with inputs such as staff numbers, qualifications and training, presence or absence of certain services; *process* indicators cover such factors as response time and patterns of client–worker interaction; and *outcome* indicators refer to the effects of services upon clients and their carers. It follows, therefore, that while indicators of outcome are the most important for assessing the effectiveness and quality of a service, they are also the most difficult and expensive to obtain. Agencies will therefore tend to use indicators of structure and process for whose validity it is necessary that a relationship between these indicators and effective outcomes is either known or reasonably presumed.

Case management agencies have begun to develop standards for practice, which are usually indicators of structure and process, and it is instructive to examine some of these. The case management standards developed by the State of Washington (1986) offer examples of several structural indicators. These include suitable office accommodation to permit private interviewing, administrative minimum standards, and case management staff possessing a relevant degree with two years experience of providing services. The same document includes such process standards as eligibility criteria for entry, a maximum caseload size of fifty, frequency of supervision, ongoing training of forty hours per year, speed of response to a referral and time taken to commence assessment and develop care plans, review periods and the maintenance of records. These are similar to the proposed standards developed by the National Institute of Community-Based Long-Term Care (1988). Additionally, in terms of outcomes the proposed national US standards include questions such as whether care plans are designed to provide adequate and appropriate services in a cost-effective manner and whether the services provided meet client need (ibid.).

Applebaum and Austin (1990) suggest five broad quality assurance questions that can be pursued once standards have been agreed and made explicit:

1. How well are eligibility and targeting criteria implemented?
2. Are assessments and care plans completed in sufficient time?
3. Do service plans meet clients' needs?
4. Are service plans actually implemented?
5. Are clients satisfied with the care received?

These bear some similarity to the different components of efficiency in Challis and Davies (1986) and cited in the Department of Health's (1991a) guidance for managers. As a quality assurance mechanism, these can be tackled in a number of ways. First, eligibility and targeting could be monitored by examination of data on the characteristics of the population of service users, possibly comparing variations between geographical areas. Independent reviews of a sample of cases would assist in validation and the use of multidisciplinary assessment could contribute to a greater standardization of judgement. The second question, developing measures of effective response time to assessment and care plans, is dependent upon the formulation of normative standards coupled with regular and independent audit and review of records. In some cases, this might be coupled with direct observation of practice. The third question, the extent to which care plans actually meet needs, is obviously an area of professional judgement. One possible approach might be the use of peer review, whether on a home visit or case record basis, and another might be the use of independent audit. A monitoring strategy, used in some US states, involves examining the degree of variation found in care plans. This is based on the proposition that care plans are meant to reflect the wide variety of individual circumstances and therefore lack of variety might be indicative of poor-quality practice. Questions about outcome such as hospital and nursing home placement could also act as relevant performance measures. The fourth question, whether or not care plans are in fact implemented, could be monitored by an analysis of individual case records and also independent audit or review of the system. The fifth question, client or carer satisfaction, has always proved a problematic area for assessment. Surveys of older people have frequently revealed high degrees of satisfaction without generating more substantively useful information. One use of surveys might be on a comparative basis, across time or teams of staff, since the pattern of variation would be a subject worthy of further investigation. An interesting technique used in one US state is for a random sample of clients and carers to be visited by independent assessors and senior managers to ask questions about service quality. Certainly this approach appears to have enhanced senior managers' appreciation of the problems of day-to-day service provision.

Logical coherence of care management arrangements

As we discussed earlier, the managerial, agency and funding environment within which such practice takes place will tend to determine what is perceived as possible and reasonable solutions to meeting need. Dant and Gearing (1990: 344) note the conclusion of many observers of the US scene: 'Case Management (alone) cannot produce coordinated care, a necessary pre-requisite is the integration of funding sources'. More broadly, four elements need to be coordinated in a fully coordinated system: programmes, resources, clients and information (Aiken *et al.*, 1975). Some programmes attempt to tackle this integration. The Manitoba Continuing Care Programme Policy Guidelines (1991) link philosophy, objectives and principles with detailed features of administration and operation. The Madison Mental Health Service illustrates clearly how the practice environment and perceptions of what is possible are influenced by the context of funding. The goals of the service are linked through organizational principles to clinical principles to offer a complete system of care (Stein and Test, 1985; Stein *et al*, 1989). Ethical factors are important too (Kane, 1988b). Hence, practice *content* is likely to be determined by the nature of the practice *context*, and a tendency to discuss case management at the level of practice content alone (Fisher, 1991) can only provide a partial understanding of the forces at work. Contextual factors such as degree of managerial support for the development, which agency employs the case managers, their span and degree of budgetary control, where they are located and what choice of target population is made will again influence the content of what case managers see as realistic and viable choices. The effective implementation of a case management model requires a coherent logic which clarifies the relationship between structure, location, target group, practice model and likely day-to-day pressures and incentives with expected outcomes.

Several of the case management studies referred to in Table 1, either directly or indirectly raise the issue of internal logical coherence – a relationship between values, desired outcomes or goals, and the practice and managerial incentives arising from structures and resources. The factors discussed earlier are all interlinked; for example, targeting policy influences caseloads, which in turn influence feasible styles of the case management process. This final point of logical coherence is also relevant to the interrelationship of systems. As the Department of Health (1990) policy guidance makes clear, there is a distinction between 'intensive case management' as discussed in this chapter and the generalization of a 'care management approach' across the service system: 'What authorities and agencies face in generalising care management to all users is not the development of one model but a range of different models, suited to the type and level of users needs'.

The analysis of the logical coherence of case management programmes should be of concern to managers and planners in reviewing the development and performance of care management in their service systems.

Conclusion

In the UK, assessment and care management have been identified as the cornerstones of a policy which is directed to achieve a degree of 'downward substitution' at the margin between settings. This reflects the view that some people require less intensive levels of care than that provided in the care setting in which they are located, and that it is more cost-effective for them to be supported in a less dependent setting (Challis, 1992c). The effective implementation of such a policy depends in particular upon the effective management of the interface between institutional and home-based care, through screening and provision of intensive home care, where both assessment and care management are critical. Indeed, the possible consequences of poor practice in this area could lead to a growth in institutional placements with the funding for home care being transferred to pay for this – the converse of a policy of community care. Hence a great deal is dependent upon the implementation of policy at the practice level and therefore upon the training, staff skills and resources available to those undertaking the work. The link between policy goals and style of practice can clearly be made.

Hence implicit within the development of care management is an expectation of a greater focus of work upon specific client groups. Much concern has been expressed about the need to train potential case managers about aspects of budgets, cost containment and associated information systems. However, it would seem unwise to see this as the only area of knowledge required. Together with the development of specialization and generally heightened awareness of community care issues, will arise legitimate expectations from the users of services for case managers to have specific knowledge about the needs, problems and service requirements of their particular client group. For the practice of effective care management it would be unwise to ignore this expectation and there will be a need to provide further skills and knowledge in these 'clinical' areas if the risk of a poorer quality brokerage model is to be avoided. The adequate resourcing of devolved budgets will also be important if perverse practice incentives are to be avoided and, given resource scarcity, this will be dependent upon how targeting is managed.

The implementation of case management is likely to be a slow process, involving the trial of different approaches in different contexts. If the experience elsewhere offers us guidance, the debate about the relative virtues of different forms and models will continue. Case management is no panacea (Hunter, 1988; Callahan, 1989), but rather a mechanism which, if effectively implemented, can offer one way to manage the tension between social objectives and economic constraints in care services, and this can never be a comfortable process. The elements discussed here cover some of the critical areas which need to be addressed if the process of implementation is to begin to achieve the desired goals for community care.

References

Aiken, M., Dewar, R., DiTomaso, N., Hager, J. and Zeitz, G. (1975). *Coordinating Human Services.* San Francisco, CA: Jossey-Bass.

Applebaum, R. and Austin, C. (1990). *Long Term Care Case Management: Design and Evaluation.* New York: Springer.

Arnold, D. (1987). The brokerage model of long term care: A rose by another name. *Home Health Care Services Quarterly,* 8(2): 23–43.

Audit Commission (1992a). *The Community Revolution: Personal Social Services and Community Care.* London: HMSO.

Audit Commission (1992b). *Community Care: Managing the Cascade of Change.* London: HMSO.

Austin, C. (1981). Client assessment in context. *Social Work Research and Abstracts,* *20*: 4–12.

Austin, C. (1983). Case management in long-term care: Options and opportunities. *Health and Social Work,* *8*(1): 16–30.

Austin, C. (1992). When the whole is more than the sum of its parts: Case management issues from a systems perspective. Paper presented at the *First International Conference on Long Term Care Case Management,* Seattle, WA.

Bachrach, L. (1992). Case management revisited. *Hospital and Community Psychiatry,* *43*: 209–210.

Ballew, J. and Mink, G. (1986). *Case Management in the Human Services.* Springfield, IL: Charles C. Thomas.

British Columbia Ministry of Health (1992). *Case Manager Guidebook.* Victoria, BC: Ministry of Health, Continuing Care Division.

Callahan, J. (1989). Case management for the elderly: A panacea? *Journal of Ageing and Social Policy,* *1*: 181–95.

Capitman, J.A., Haskins, B. and Bernstein, J. (1986). Case management approaches in community-oriented long term care demonstrations. *The Gerontologist,* *26*: 398–404.

Challis, D. (1992a). The care of the elderly in Europe: New directions – social care. *European Journal of Gerontology,* *1*: 334–47.

Challis, D. (1992b). Community care of elderly people: Bringing together scarcity and choice, needs and costs. *Financial Accountability and Management,* *8*: 77–95.

Challis, D. (1992c). Providing alternatives to long stay hospital care for frail elderly patients: Is it cost effective? *International Journal of Geriatric Psychiatry,* *7*: 773–81.

Challis, D. and Davies, B. (1985). Long term care for the elderly: The community care scheme. *British Journal of Social Work,* *15*: 563–79.

Challis, D. and Davies, B. (1986). *Case Management in Community Care.* Aldershot: Gower.

Challis, D., Chessum, R., Chesterman, J., Luckett, R. and Woods, B. (1988). Community care for the frail elderly: An urban experiment. *British Journal of Social Work,* *18*: 43–54 (suppl.).

Challis, D., Darton, R., Johnson, L., Stone, M., Traske, K. and Wall, B. (1989). *Supporting Frail Elderly People at Home: The Darlington Community Care Project.* Canterbury: Personal Social Services Research Unit, University of Kent.

Challis, D., Chessum, R., Chesterman, J., Luckett, R. and Traske, K. (1990). *Case Management in Social and Health Care.* Canterbury: Personal Social Services Research Unit, University of Kent.

Challis, D., Darton, R., Johnson, L., Stone, M. and Traske, K. (1991a). An evaluation of an alternative to long-stay hospital care for frail elderly patients. Part I: The model of care. *Age and Ageing,* *20*: 236–44.

Challis, D., Darton, R., Johnson, L., Stone, M. and Traske, K. (1991b). An evaluation of an alternative to long-stay hospital care for the frail elderly. Part II: Costs and outcomes. *Age and Ageing,* *20*: 245–54.

Challis, D., Chessum, R., Chesterman, J., Luckett, R. and Traske, K. (1992). Case management in health and social care. In Lazcko, F. and Victor, C. (eds), *Social Policy and Elderly People.* Aldershot: Avebury/Gower.

Challis, D., Chesterman, J., Darton, R. and Traske, K. (1993). Case management in the care of the aged: The provision of care in different settings. In Barnett, J., Pereira, C., Pilgrim, D. and Williams, F. (eds), *Community Care: A Reader*. Basingstoke: Macmillan.

Chamberlain, R. and Rapp, C.A. (1991). A decade of case management: A methodological review of outcome research. *Community Mental Journal, 27*: 171–88.

Community Options Programme (1992). *Community Options Programme: Guidelines and Procedures*. Madison, WI: Department of Health and Social Services.

Dant, T. and Gearing, B. (1990). Keyworkers for elderly people in the community: Case managers and care coordinators. *Journal of Social Policy, 19*: 331–60.

Dant, T., Carley, M., Gearing, B. and Johnson, M. (1989). *Coordinating Car: Final Report of the Care for the Elderly People at Home Project*. Milton Keynes/London: Open University/Policy Studies Institute.

Davies, B. and Challis, D. (1986). *Matching Resources to Needs in Community Care*. Aldershot: Gower.

Department of Health (1989). *Caring for People: Community Care in the Next Decade and Beyond*. Cm. 849. London: HMSO.

Department of Health (1990). *Caring for People: Community Care in the Next Decade and Beyond. Policy Guidance*. London: HMSO.

Department of Health (1991a). *Care Management and Assessment: Manager's Guide*. London: HMSO.

Department of Health (1991b). *Care Management and Assessment: Practitioner's Guide*. London: HMSO.

Department of Health and Social Security (1983). *Care in the Community*. HC(83)6, LAC(83)5. London: HMSO.

Donabedian, A. (1980). *The Definition of Quality and Approaches to its Assessment*. Ann Arbor, Mich.: Health Administration Press.

Financial Management Partnership (1992). *Statement of User Requirements for the Financial Management of Community Care*. London: CIPFA.

Fineman, L. (1992). A community care system for the elderly in Manitoba, Canada. Paper presented at the *International Symposium on Social Care for the Elderly: Community Care Systems in the Human Services*, Tokyo.

Fisher, M. (1991). Defining the practice content of case management. *Social Work and Social Science Review, 2*: 204–230.

Gregory, R. (1991). *Aged Care Reform Strategy: Mid Term Review 1990–91*. Canberra: Australian Government Publishing Service.

Griffiths, R. (1988). *Community Care: Agenda for Action*. London: HMSO.

Harris, M. and Bachrach, L. (eds) (1988). *Clinical Case Management*. New Directions for Mental Health Services No. 40. San Francisco, CA: Jossey-Bass.

Harris, M. and Bergman, H. (1987). Case management with the chronically mentally ill: A clinical perspective. *American Journal of Orthopsychiatry, 57*: 296–302.

Hennessy, C. and Hennessy, M. (1990). Community-based long term care for the elderly: Evaluation and practice reconsidered. *Medical Care Review, 47*: 221–59.

Hoult, J. (1990). Dissemination in New South Wales of the Madison model. In Marks, I. and Scott, R. (eds), *Mental Health Care Delivery: Innovation, Impediment and Implementation*. Cambridge: Cambridge University Press.

Hoult, J., Reynolds, I., Charbonneau-Powis, M., Weekes, P. and Briggs, J. (1983).

Psychiatric hospital versus community treatment: The results of a randomised trial. *Australian and New Zealand Journal of Psychiatry, 17*: 160–67.

Hunter, D. (1988). Managed care: The problem and the remedy. In Hunter, D. (ed.), *Bridging the Gap: Case Management and Advocacy for People with Physical Handicaps.* London: King's Fund.

Huxley, P. (1991). Effective case management for mentally ill people: The relevance of recent evidence from the USA for case management services in the United Kingdom. *Social Work and Social Science Review, 2*: 192–203.

Huxley, P., Hagan, T., Hennelly, R. and Hunt, J. (1990). *Effective Community Mental Health Services.* Aldershot: Avebury/Gower.

Intagliata, J. (1982). Improving the quality of community care for the chronically mentally disabled: The role of case management. *Schizophrenia Bulletin, 8*: 655–74.

Kane, R. (1988a). The noblest experiment of them all: Learning from the National Channelling Evaluation. *Health Services Research, 23*(1): 189–98.

Kane, R. (1988b). Case management: Ethical pitfalls on the road to high quality managed care. *Quality Review Bulletin, 14*: 161–6.

Kane, R. (1990). *What is Case Management Anyway?* Minneapolis: Long-term Care Decisions Resource Center, University of Minnesota.

Kane, R. and Kane, R. (1991). Home and community based care in Canada. In Rowland, D. and Lyons, B. (eds), *Financing Home Care: Improving Protection for Disabled Elderly People.* Baltimore, MD: Johns Hopkins University Press.

Kanter, J. (1987). Mental health case management: A professional domain? *Social Work, 32*: 461–2.

Kanter, J. (1989). Clinical case management: Definition, principles, components. *Hospital and Community Psychiatry, 40*: 361–8.

Kemper, P. (1988). The evaluation of the National Long Term Care Demonstration: 10. Overview of the findings. *Health Services Research, 23*: 161–73.

Kraan, R.J., Baldock, J., Davies, B., Evers, A., Johansson, L., Knapen, M., Thorslund, M. and Tunissen, C. (1991). *Care for the Elderly: Significant Innovations in Three European Countries.* Boulder, CO: Campus/Westview.

Liu, K. and Cornelius, E. (1991). Activities of daily living and eligibility for home care. In Rowland, D. and Lyons, B. (eds), *Financing Home Care: Improving Protection for Disabled Elderly People.* Baltimore, MD: Johns Hopkins University Press.

Luehrs, J. and Ramthun, R. (1991). State approaches to functional assessments for home care. In Rowland, D. and Lyons, B. (eds), *Financing Home Care: Improving Protection for Disabled Elderly People.* Baltimore, MD: Johns Hopkins University Press.

Lutz, B. (1989). *Report of Development and Testing of Screening and Assessment Instruments.* Paper No. 12. Stirling: Social Work Research Centre, University of Stirling.

McDowell, D., Barniskis, L. and Wright, S. (1990). The Wisconsin Community Options Programme: Planning and packaging long-term support for individuals. In Howe, A., Ozanne, E. and Selby Smith, C. (eds), *Community Care Policy and Practice: New Directions in Australia.* Victoria: Public Sector Management Institute, Monash University.

Manitoba Department of Health (1991). *Policy Guidelines: Continuing Care.* Winnipeg, Manitoba: Department of Health.

Miller, G. (1983). Case management: The essential service. In Sanborn, C. (ed.), *Case Management in Mental Health Services*. New York: Haworth Press.

Modricin, M., Rapp, C. and Poertner, J. (1988). The evaluation of case management services with the chronically mentally ill. *Evaluation and Programme Planning, 11*: 307–314.

Moore, S.T. (1990). A social work practice model of case management: The case management grid. *Social Work, 35*: 444–8.

Moxley, D. (1989). *The Practice of Case Management*. Newbury Park, CA: Sage.

National Development Team (1991). *The Andover Case Management Project*. London: NDT.

National Institute of Community-Based Long-Term Care (1988). *Care Management Standards: Guidelines for Practice*. Washington, DC: NICBLTC, National Institute of Ageing.

Neill, J., Sinclair, I., Gorbach, P. and Williams, J. (1988). *A Need for Care: Elderly Applicants for Local Authority Homes*. Aldershot: Avebury/Gower.

O'Connor, G. (1988). Case management: System and practice. *Social Casework, 69*: 97–106.

Pilling, D. (1988). *The Case Manager Project: Report of the Evaluation*. London: Rehabilitation Resource Centre, City University.

Pilling, D. (1992). *Approaches to Case Management for People with Disabilities*. London: Jessica Kingsley.

Richardson, A. and Higgins, R. (1990). *Case Management in Practice: Reflections on the Wakefield Case Management Project*. Working Paper No. 1. Leeds: Nuffield Institute for Health Service Studies, University of Leeds.

Richardson, A. and Higgins, R. (1992). *The Limits of Case Management: Lessons from the Wakefield Case Management Project*. Working Paper No. 5. Leeds: Nuffield Institute for Health Service Studies, University of Leeds.

Roberts-DeGennaro, M. (1987). Defining case management as a practice model. *Social Casework, 68*: 466–70.

Rothman, J (1991). A model of case management: Toward empirically based practice. *Social Work, 36*: 520–28.

Stein, L.I. (1989). *Wisconsin's System of Mental Health Financing*. Madison, WI: Mental Health Research Center, University of Wisconsin.

Stein, L.I. and Test, M.A. (1980). Alternative to mental hospital treatment: I. Conceptual model, treatment programme, and clinical evaluation. *Archives of General Psychiatry, 37*: 392–7.

Stein, L.I. and Test, M.A. (1985). The evolution of the training in community living model. In Stein, L.I. and Test, M.A. (eds), *The Training in Community Living Model: A Decade of Experience*. New Directions in Mental Health Service No. 26. San Francisco, CA: Jossey-Bass.

Stein, L.I., Diamond, R. and Factor, R. (1989). *A System Approach to the Care of Persons with Schizophrenia*. Madison, WI: Mental Health Research Center, University of Wisconsin.

Steinberg, R.M. and Carter, G.W. (1983). *Case Management and the Elderly*. Lexington, MA: Heath.

Test, M.A. and Stein, L.I. (1980). Alternative to mental hospital treatment: III. Social cost. *Archives of General Psychiatry, 37*: 409–412.

Washington State (1986). *Information and Assistance/Case Management Standards.* Olympia, WA: Department of Social and Health Services.

Weisbrod, B., Test, M.A. and Stein, L.I. (1980). Alternative to mental hospital treatment: II. Economic benefit cost analysis. *Archives of General Psychiatry, 37*: 400–405.

Weissert, G. (1988). The National Channelling Demonstration: What we knew, know now and still need to know. *Health Services Research, 23*: 175–87.

Section 2

Staff and users

5 The caring professions

John Brown

The passing by Parliament of the NHS and Community Care Act 1990 marked a significant shift in the provision and delivery of community care offered by statutory and independent agencies. Specific aspects of the legislation were not introduced immediately so that, for example, social services led responsibility for community care was delayed until April 1993. However, the White Papers upon which the legislation was based incorporated statements that were to set the agenda for detailed debate on a variety of topics at local level. Foremost among these topics was the issue of training staff to meet the needs of clients as the new structures of service delivery were planned and implemented.

In the 1989 White Paper, *Caring for People: Community Care in the Next Decade and Beyond*, a firm commitment was made by the government to multidisciplinary training as an essential approach to staffing the services of the 1990s: 'It will be important to continue to develop multidisciplinary training for staff in all caring professions including the provision of joint training at both the qualifying and post-qualifying stages' (Department of Health, 1989b: 67). Multidisciplinary training, or 'shared learning' as it is increasingly coming to be called (CCETSW, 1992; UKCC, 1992), provides the focus for this chapter. While the issues identified apply specifically to shared learning, the issues they raise provide an indication of the range of topics that the caring professions as a whole have to address as services evolve in the 1990s. Similarly, while shared learning has made great inroads in the development of collaborative links between nursing and social work, the lessons have application to all occupational groups identified within the phrase 'the caring professions'. These collaborative developments have had most impact on staff training in learning disabilities.

In 1990, one year after the publication of *Caring for People*, a Training Strategy Group was established, jointly chaired by the Social Services Inspectorate and the Central Council for Education and Training in Social Work (CCETSW), which took forward joint training at six sites throughout

England (DoH/SSI, 1991). Although the initiative focused upon the elderly and people with a mental illness, joint training had made greatest progress at that time in the field of learning disabilities. Despite a hesitant, and at times acrimonious, start in the early 1980s, a number of joint and shared programmes were underway in learning disabilities as the Training Strategy Group started its work (Brown, 1992). Such developments indicate that activities often at the margin of professional interest, a position occupied by learning disabilities in both social work and nursing, can often respond to changing policy imperatives with a speed that is not possible for the mainstream of a profession.

If there is one general observation to be made about the cumulative impact of health and community care initiatives from the mid-1980s onwards, it is of the pace and volume of change. Learning disabilities, on the fringes of professional priorities, could respond to change quickly. Shared learning is very much a manifestation of this response and provides a barometer for predicting changing conditions that will affect all those working within the caring professions.

This chapter is divided into two sections. In the first, 'The contractual environment', a number of issues are identified that provide the current policy context for professional practice and training. The second, 'Implementing local innovation', specifically focuses upon shared learning. Steps in the process of implementation are identified that reflect aspects of introducing innovation in the way that the caring professions prepare their staff.

The contractual environment

For thirty years, ever since the legislation of the mid- to late 1940s laid the foundations for the Welfare State, there was a general consensus over, and commitment to, the values of welfare and the responsibilities of the state. This consensus provided the policy parameters within which the caring professions carried out their practice. In 1979, with the election of a Conservative government, this consensus was shattered by the ascendance of a New Right ideology that questioned, among many items, levels of public expenditure and occupational demarcation. In the 1990s, there is now a clear set of new policy parameters that set the agenda for the caring professions and reflect a clear legacy of the Thatcher years. Symbolically, the year that Thatcher was deposed, 1990, was also the year that the new National Health Service (NHS) and community care legislation was passed onto the statute book.

In 1989, the two White Papers *Working for Patients* and *Caring for People* (Department of Health, 1989a, 1989b), together with *Promoting Better Health*

(DHSS, 1987), formed the basis of the NHS and Community Care Act 1990. Ever since the initial community care plans of the early 1960s, there had been controversy and confusion over lead-agency responsibility for community care. The legislation resolved this debate of three decades by identifying clear lead responsibility with social services. The first impact of the 1990 Act, however, was to be found in health, and nursing, as the timetable for introducing the legislation delayed the full implementation of the community care proposals until April 1993.

As health and social services are having to respond to the same pressures, the experiences within health have begun to provide directions for activities within local government. In particular, the essentials of the 'general management function', originally introduced after the 1983 Griffiths Enquiry, have been incorporated into government plans for restructuring the way that local government functions (Department of Environment, 1991). At the same time, the purchaser–provider split, essential to the new approach to providing community care (Department of Health, 1989a, 1990), has already been introduced in health with the formation of self-governing trust hospitals.

The impact of initiatives such as these is all part of an emerging contractual environment that, following statements in *Working for Patients* and *Caring for People, must* be based upon the identified needs of the client. Traditional patterns of service provision and training programmes are not sacrosanct. They must be shown to meet the needs of the client by any of the current means of evaluating outcomes, especially those related to assessing 'quality'. This is but one of a number of discernible trends that reflect the new policy parameters.

Commissioning agencies

The purchaser–provider split is essential to the internal market already underway in the NHS and about to be introduced in social services. The contracts that define the relationship between agencies are still very much an area of intense discussion regarding the negotiation procedure, detailed content, monitoring procedures and outcome measures. In the training agenda, the issue is very much how client needs are assessed and the ways that the skills identified to meet these needs inform training programmes. Within shared learning, the focus has been upon the balance and emphasis of skills contributed by different occupational groups – and how these are incorporated into contracts.

In particular, emphasis is placed upon drawing up contracts based upon a client needs analysis that identifies skills required from shared learning. Professional training, as well as practice, is now increasingly being defined and incorporated into explicit contracts of performance and outcome.

Local ownership

Services and training programmes are increasingly being seen as local initiatives that are designed specifically to meet the requirements of the local setting. Along with this goes the feeling of 'local ownership'. There is the beginning of a discernible trend for local managers to develop their own specific training courses rather than patronize courses offering a regional, if not national, expertise. A key issue that this raises is comparability in standards between courses in different localities. This is given added impetus with proposed changes in CCETSW and new roles for the ENB emphasizing the importance of national criteria upon which standards can be evaluated. For service provision, guidelines have been published on standards for residential care, although mechanisms for comparison still need to be established (DoH/SSI, 1993). For training programmes, developments in National Vocational Qualifications (NVQ) provide one way forward (Joint Awarding Bodies, 1990).

The caring professions are now faced with attempts to determine the criteria and mechanisms required for ensuring comparability between locally based initiatives. The role of identifying, and enforcing, national standards in the local setting is still very much in its early stages.

Employer-led training

A distinctive trend in the late 1980s and early 1990s has been the emergence of employer-led training to challenge the historical predominance of profession-determined education. The involvement of employers at a regional level in Training and Enterprise Councils (TECs) is mirrored with their involvement in specific programmes such as BTEC Diplomas and ACCESS courses. Employers are increasingly being involved and integrated within the Diploma in Social Work as they are in health service training.

Alternative qualifications to those offered by the professions are emerging and a national criteria of comparison has been developed with the work on NVQs. Although social work has been actively involved in discussions about the content of specific competence levels, nursing has been much more ambivalent. Reluctance to be involved in the Care Sector Consortium has been reflected in the rejection of direct involvement in the work of the Joint Awarding Bodies. This has been extended to a decision not to be party to discussions on the development of occupational standards.

Despite the antipathy of the nursing profession to contribute to the development of competence-based training, it is clear, nonetheless, that 'competence' as promulgated by the National Council of Vocational Qualifications is the currency in which all future training programmes will have to be expressed. Shared learning is no exception. Professional training has to be integrated within the range of competence as defined by NVQ occupational standards from the most simple through to the most advanced activity. It is no longer possible to discuss professional preparation divorced from the needs of all the workforce.

Multidisciplinary mix

Multidisciplinary training is being actively promoted by central government – and not only in the several White Papers in the late 1980s, but also in documents with a more specific focus. For example, the Tomlinson Report (Department of Health, 1992) on health services in London advocated multidisciplinary training for medical practitioners at both the undergraduate and postgraduate levels. The multidisciplinary 'mix' highlights issues of demarcation between occupational groups that shared learning explicitly recognizes. At the same time, shared learning begins to 'blur' boundaries in a way that parallels the arguments for a seamless service (Audit Commission, 1992a, 1992b, 1992c). Contemporary arguments for developing services assume that traditional boundaries are no longer appropriate; shared learning is a potential vehicle for redefining those boundaries. The contribution of shared learning to the multidisciplinary mix, however, is still far from certain.

Appraisal

Self-governing trusts within the NHS have the legislative framework through which they can negotiate individual salaries, independent of National Pay Reviews and Whitley Council levels, for all staff including clinicians. A development such as this is becoming an integral part of staff appraisal – annual performance reviews, discretionary payments and the like – and there is a move towards short-term contracts renewable (or otherwise) on an annual basis. Terms and conditions of employment are undergoing significant changes. Shared learning programmes cannot be divorced from the employment context faced by successful students. Appraisal systems, in particular, have to address the particular cluster of skills such students bring to their organizational tasks. This is a development that highlights how changes in service infrastructure have also to be considered in tandem with changes in employment terms and conditions. The caring professions are facing potential new patterns of employment that will have a direct impact upon their practice.

Management function

Managers in health, and increasingly in social services, are employed on short-term contracts. The renewal of such contracts requires set performance targets to be met. The pursuit of these targets, and the style adopted, plays a significant role in establishing an organizational ambience in which staff practice is undertaken. The line-management structure itself determines the level of support, and the degree of 'risk' tolerated, which staff experience. The impact of managerialism in the public sector is a crucial element in determining whether students from shared learning programmes are allowed to realize their potential contribution.

As a corollary, an issue to be addressed is whether such students can promote change within an organization when, as relatively junior members of the team (albeit with the possibility of 'fast-track' promotion), they do not have the organizational weight to take the appropriate responsibility. Line-management support, at all levels, is critical if shared learning is to help initiate as well as reinforce change within an organization.

Information technology

Ever since the Körner initiatives in the early 1980s, the NHS has gathered information of an ever increasing complexity. Although the question arises 'information for what purpose?', there is no denying that manpower exercises on recruitment, retention, projected demands and the like have evolved into detailed workforce planning exercises. These exercises are an essential source of information for managers to base decisions on.

Any exercise in workforce planning has to gather appropriate information upon which to analyse the current situation and anticipate possible trends. For staffing projections it is essential to assess likely career patterns and, as services strive to become seamless, possible paths of staff mobility within and across agencies. It is still not clear what the career paths are likely to be in the future. But for shared learning to consolidate its position in the local agenda, it is crucial to address such issues. To fail to consider broad workforce planning issues is to limit the relevance, and therefore development, of shared learning.

The seven trends, and the issues they raise, are summarized in Table 1. The elements identified reflect a number of clear activities pursued by the government in health and social care (Brown, 1994a):

- the treatment of professions as trade unions;
- the questioning of long-established patterns of demarcation;
- the establishment of a contract culture;
- the encouragement of local salary negotiations;
- the development of alternative qualifications to those recognized by the professions;
- the introduction of changes in the legislative framework; and
- the alteration of the infrastructure for service responsibilities.

Table 1 Parameters for shared learning

Trend	Issue	Focus
Commissioning agencies	Contracts	Client needs analysis determining skills required
Local ownership	National standards	Criteria and mechanisms for comparing services
Employer-led training	Competence	Programmes and qualifications within NVQ
Multidisciplinary mix	Demarcation	Integration of occupations in a seamless service
Locally negotiated salaries	Appraisal	Terms and conditions of employment
Management function	Line-management	Managerialism and staff performance
Information gathering	Workforce planning	Career profiles within and between agencies

Source: Brown (1994b).

The cumulative impact of these activities is to highlight the importance of how initiatives, involving the caring professions, are introduced and implemented in the local setting.

Implementing local innovation

Towards the end of 1991, as part of its community care initiative, the Department of Health published a paper titled *Training for Community Care: A Joint Approach* (DoH/SSI, 1991). This document took further the commitment outlined in *Caring for People* (Department of Health, 1989b) to interdisciplinary training at all levels of staff preparation. In particular, a range of operational possibilities were presented that emphasized the necessity of service purchasers and providers considering new alignments between occupational groups if the NHS and Community Care Act 1990 is to be implemented successfully. The challenge that this legislation presents for statutory and independent agencies was highlighted in early 1992 with publication by the Audit Commission of a series of reports on health and community care. In *The Cascade of Change, Homeward Bound* and *The Community Revolution,* the Audit Commission (1992a, 1992b, 1992c) itemized a detailed catalogue of issues – vision, strategic planning, care co-ordination, managing service delivery, information systems, quality assurance – faced by the NHS and local government. With lead-responsibility for community care taken over by local government in April 1993, the reports were a timely reminder of the problems that can beset the statutory and independent sectors when striving to work in new ways for the benefit of service users and clients. These problems were not unexpected.

In the early 1980s, the promotion of joint training approaches by the nursing and social work validating bodies did not meet with a receptive audience in either profession. The climate of the time meant that when two reports on qualifying and post-qualifying training were published, in 1982 and 1983 respectively, they were greeted with antipathy at best and hostility at worst from some nurses and social workers (General Nursing Councils/CCETSW, 1982, 1983). It was not until the announcement late in 1986 of a new initiative between the English National Board for Nursing, Midwifery and Health Visiting (ENB) and CCETSW that it was possible to take the debate, and tentative schemes on the ground, forward (ENB/CCETSW, 1986). The following five years marked a particularly active time when joint/shared training in learning disabilities began to make appreciable strides forward at all levels of staff preparation (Thompson and Mathias, 1992). These initiatives, which embrace all levels of training, have indicated a number of preliminary steps when caring professions are brought together under the impetus of shared learning (Brown, 1994b).

- *Agreement over, and clarity of, purpose.* Is the shared learning initiative to be used to: Increase awareness/understanding of other occupational groups' contribution to service delivery? Prepare staff to supplement the work of others and possibly, if required, take on a locum function, replace existing staff or retrain existing staff? Questions such as these have to be considered and agreement reached on precisely what the objectives are for introducing shared learning.
- *Involvement and commitment at all levels of sponsoring organizations.* Change is at the point of delivery of a service. With the increasing, and appropriate, emphasis upon management involvement, it is important not to forget the importance of carrying direct care staff along with any initiative.
- *Clear lines of responsibility.* All too often success rises up the organization, while failure sinks to lower levels. Responsibility and accountability need to be clearly identified and recognized at or towards the beginning of the introduction of an initiative.
- *Balanced representation on training programmes.* In practice, course participants are dominated by recruitment from a particular occupational group, especially nursing. This immediately raises the possibility of the largest group creating a dominant ethos that may, or may not, undermine the objective of shared learning.
- *Evolution of service structures.* Service structures have to develop and evolve in advance of, or in parallel with, training initiatives. The often stated

objective of shared training that it relates to developments in service structures can obscure the fact that such developments often fail to occur. In these circumstances, shared learning is necessary but not sufficient in itself to ensure change.

* *Flexible employment.* A flexible approach to terms and conditions of employment is required. Rigidity can dominate and undermine the employability of those who have experienced shared learning initiatives in terms of opportunities and enhanced salaries.
* *Two-way employment opportunities.* Employment opportunities can be one-way. How many social workers experience shared learning and then seek health authority employment? Shared learning often means, in reality, retraining nurses. It is important that those who organize such programmes are explicit about their objectives and the subsequent employment opportunities. It is also important to be clear about the process involved in pursuing the objectives.

The increasing emphasis upon 'outcome' and 'output', especially in training and education programmes, has tended to deflect attention away from 'process'. Process, however, is crucial and it is possible to identify a four-step process.

Definition

In the initial stages of a new initiative in shared learning, it is essential to reach agreement on objectives and procedures. There has to be a feeling of ownership among senior personnel and during the introduction of the scheme there needs to be continuity among senior staff – especially difficult given the administrative and organizational changes underway at present. The primary requirement is to identify and reach agreement over a 'sponsor'.

Design

When designing a shared learning initiative, it is essential to recognize the importance of an honest broker. Difficulties often experienced in pursuing cooperation and collaboration between different agencies can lead to problems in taking forward new initiatives. What is required is an independent 'third party' to bring together, and work with, different sectors. The 'third party' may not be independent in reality – as long as there is the perception of independence.

Delivery

It can be crucial to carry all staff with the initiative, especially those directly involved in delivering the programme. It is at this organizational

Table 2 Local implementation of shared learning

Phase	Primary role	Key element
Definition	Sponsor	Ownership by, and continuity among, senior management
Design	Broker	Independent 'third party' to bring together, and work with, different sectors
Delivery	Architect	Commitment, vision and lateral thought from course educators
Deployment	Counsellor	Support for jointly qualified staff in their practice

Source: Brown (1994b).

level that opportunities to undermine and/or sabotage shared learning initiatives can proliferate. It is essential that course educators, who in essence are the architects of course training, display commitment, vision and lateral thought. One way to encourage this is to ensure that course educators are involved at both the 'definition' and 'design' stages.

Deployment

Staff who have successfully completed shared learning can often experience difficulties in their professional identity. This is especially the case if students have been on jointly validated qualifying courses where they may not necessarily bring to the course a predominant 'nurse' or 'social worker' identity. When subsequently deployed in the organization, it may not be readily apparent how best to use their 'unique' combination of skills, leading to frustration for the practitioner. In some cases, expectations might be high that the practitioner can influence, if not initiate, change. These expectations can lead to stress for the individual who is still, generally, a junior member of staff after the course without the organizational authority to meet the employer's expectations. These, and related issues of motivation and retention, make it imperative to provide support for jointly qualified staff in their practice. The primary requirement of a 'counsellor' cannot be overemphasized.

These four stages in the process of joint qualifying training are summarized in Table 2.

A positive change?

The emergence of the 'contract culture' in the delivery of health and community care has altered both the terminology and emphasis of the services that are to be provided and purchased by the statutory and independent sectors. Shared learning, as with any initiative, has to place its priorities within the prevailing political climate.

When nurses and social workers involved with learning disabilities pioneered joint/shared training in the early 1980s, it was essentially a stopgap initiative. This has evolved over the decade to a situation where shared learning is seen by central government as possessing the potential to be a stepping-stone to new patterns of training and occupational work for the caring professions. The impact of the contractual environment means, however, that developments in the caring professions now depend upon how purchasers and providers view their activities in general and shared learning in particular.

Whether this proves to be a 'positive change' (Wagner, 1993) for the client and user of services remains to be seen.

References

Audit Commission (1992a). *Community Care: Managing the Cascade of Change.* London: HMSO.

Audit Commission (1992b). *Homeward Bound.* London: HMSO.

Audit Commission (1992c). *The Community Revolution.* London: HMSO.

Brown, J. (1992). Professional boundaries: The training debate. In Thompson, T. and Mathias, P. (eds), *Standards and Mental Handicap: Keys to Competence*, pp. 352–70. London: Baillière Tindall.

Brown, J. (1994a). Demarcation and the public sector. In Thompson, T. and Mathias, P. (eds), *Mental Health and Disorder.* London: Baillière Tindall, pp. 573–586.

Brown, J. (1994b). *The Hybrid Worker.* London: CCETSW/SPSW Publishing.

CCETSW (1992). *Learning Together: Shaping New Services for People with Learning Disabilities.* Developing Partnerships in the Caring Professions No. 1. London: CCETSW.

CCETSW/ENB (1986). *Cooperation in Qualifying and Post-qualifying Training: Mental Handicap.* Report of the ENB/CCETSW Joint Working Group. London: CCETSW/ENB.

Department of Environment (1991). *The Internal Management of Local Authorities: A Consultation Paper.* London: HMSO.

Department of Health (1989a). *Working for Patients.* Cm. 555. London: HMSO.

Department of Health (1989b). *Caring for People: Community Care in the Next Decade and Beyond.* Cm. 849. London: HMSO.

Department of Health (1990). *Caring for People: Policy Guidance.* London: HMSO.

Department of Health (1992). *Report of the Inquiry into London's Health Service, Medical Education and Research.* The Tomlinson Report. London: HMSO.

Department of Health and Social Security (1987). *Promoting Better Health.* Cm. 249. London: HMSO.

Department of Health/Social Services Inspectorate (1991). *Training for Community Care: A Joint Approach.* London: HMSO.

Department of Health/Social Services Inspectorate (1993). *Guidance on Standards for the Residential Care Needs of People with Learning Disabilities/Mental Handicap.* London: HMSO.

General Nursing Councils/CCETSW (1982). *Cooperation in Training Part 1: Qualifying Training.* London: GNCs/CCETSW.

General Nursing Councils/CCETSW (1983). *Cooperation in Training Part 2: Inservice Training.* London: GNCs/CCETSW.

Griffiths, R. (1983). *NHS Management Inquiry.* London: DHSS.

Joint Awarding Bodies (1990). *Introduction of National Vocational Qualifications in Social Care and Health Care.* London: JAB.

Thompson, T. and Mathias, P. (eds) (1992). *Standards in Mental Handicap: Keys to Competence.* London: Baillière Tindall.

UKCC (1992). *Shared Learning.* Registrar's Letter 28. London: UK Central Council for Nursing, Midwifery and Health Visiting.

Wagner, G. (1993). *Residential Care – Positive Answers.* London: HMSO.

6 The family and informal care

Jill Manthorpe

Introduction

There are probably still some computers with a spell check facility that if the word 'carer' is entered, rejects it and suggest the word 'career' instead. This illustrates two things: first, the novelty of the word 'carer', it not being part of normal vocabulary until recently; and, second, that although it may be part of professional welfare language, it is unlikely yet to be commonly accepted and used, and is still open to misinterpretation.

This chapter is concerned with informal care, namely regular physical or personal assistance to people with disabilities or illness by people who are not paid to provide such assistance. This is a very broad definition and is somewhat superficial. However, it is a working definition with which we can start to consider the realities of informal care in Britain today. This chapter is organized in three main sections, looking first at demographic issues such as who does what to whom. We then discuss policy and professional responses to carers and carers' responses to these. Lastly, we look at some of the major assumptions behind informal care. The focus of this chapter is on carers who are supporting another adult, although clearly some of these adults may have been, or still are, the children of the carers. Naturally, there are many interconnections in caring for people of whatever age, but readers are referred to other texts if they wish to pursue this aspect further in relation to children.

Demographic details

Research on informal care has had a chequered and curious career in the UK. It is a mixture of small-scale research studies, of biography, of pressure-group literature and of specific description centred around a disease or medical condition. Much research on the care of disabled children permeates the debates on informal care generally, combined with a sprinkling of anthropological/sociological research into broad community networks. Bringing this into a coherent whole has been the challenge for researchers in the 1980s and, to a large extent, this has been done in the UK with studies that address the 'who does what' aspects coupled with research that considers the experience of caring.

Twigg *et al.* (1990) note that research characterizes carers in a variety of forms:

- by their *own* characteristics (e.g., age, race, gender, class);
- by the characteristics of the person being cared *for* (e.g. dementia, or physical condition);
- by their *relationship* to the person being cared for (e.g. daughter, spouse, child).

By examining these characteristics and particularly by linking such factors, we can attempt to make sense of a complex world.

The most important piece of extant research is the 1985 General Household Survey (GHS; Green, 1988), which provides new data on the prevalence of informal care in Britain. Its findings are significant in noting the size of the caring population (six million people), in drawing attention to spouse carers, particularly men, and identifying the numbers of people who were living with the person they looked after (1.7 million) and the numbers who were spending at least twenty hours each week on caring tasks (1.4 million).

As Parker (1992: 9) comments, there are at least two different sorts of caring activity which can be identified from the GHS report and which have different implications for service providers. Among the six million carers are 'People who are substantially involved, providing personal and physical care, as well as many other types of assistance, in their own household and for long hours' (ibid.: p. 14). We may term these carers as being substantially or heavily involved; no doubt another term will evolve. The other group of carers Parker terms informal helpers: 'They provide practical help to friends, neighbours, and less close relatives, who do not live in the same household, and for relatively few hours' (ibid.: p. 14). This division among the lines of activity naturally interconnects with factors such as household arrangements, relationships and economic factors. It is useful however in focusing on what people do.

Such a focus of course does not deny that there are enormous differences between carers and their experiences. We can briefly focus on these to highlight the dynamic nature of the relationship. Caring takes place in a context and chief in that context is the person who receives support or assistance. Again we are hampered by a lack of appropriate vocabulary to describe the recipient of informal care.

Similarities and differences – the gender debate

A key aspect in the political discovery of carers (see below) has been the voice of women, often expressed collectively through the feminist movement. There exists a substantial theoretical debate about the role of women in providing care influenced by many accounts of the experiences of women carers (e.g. Biggs and Oliver, 1985). It is commonly pointed out that women have a significant role as carers and are most likely to receive care (because of increasing longevity and likelihood of living alone) as well as being the main providers of care from formal organizations (Brown and Smith, 1992). There is therefore an interweaving of factors over space, place and time.

In this section, we look at two main issues. First, we explore the influence of the archetypal single woman as both a role model and influential stereotype for policy and professional service delivery. Second, we examine Ungerson's (1987: 2) claim that sex and gender do make a difference in the community care structures and processes, tying this to debates about male carers and family policy.

The spinster model

The single woman caring for her elderly frail parents has a long social history and is frequently portrayed in the literature. She may have foresaken a career, marriage and thus children, and may face a lifetime of domestic nursing followed by a lonely and impoverished old age. The White Paper, *Growing Older* (DHSS, 1981), acknowledges the martyrdom of such women. Their care and support '. . . may often involve considerable personal sacrifice, particularly where the "family" is one person, often a single woman, caring for an elderly relative' (para. 6.7, p. 37). As Finch and Mason (1993) describe it, this role would have been negotiated and is tied up with complicated ideas about reputation and moral identity. The spinster model affected policy in two important ways. The first was financial, in that such social security and allied provision that exists for carers was built on the notion that women would need a replacement wage if single, would need their pension rights protecting and would need to be excused strenuous tests of seeking work once their relatives died in order to receive income support. Associated with this have been arguments in the field of housing to allow carers to succeed to tenancies.

Second, the 'spinster model' gave an overwhelming picture of caring as women's work. It later grew to encompass married women, but these two were stereotyped as being of the same generational cohort, to have given up work or to be torn between competing demands and to be involved in caring for parent(s) or parent(s) in law. The spinster and the housewife have become entwined. This focuses attention on their similarities as daughters but neglects other important issues, such as whether people live together, whether there are reciprocal benefits that are either contemporaneous or historical, and whether care is provided at the heavy end or as informal support to a lesser extent.

Sex and gender

With such a stereotype the issue of gender has become crucial in debates about community care policy and practice. Indeed, because of the spinster legacy, it has always been important if understated, particularly in government policy documents. In the 1980s, the role stereotypes of spinsters, housewives and mothers began to coalesce into discussions about the gendered nature of community care. Influential studies from feminist writers played a key part in these developments. Land (1991), for example, questions whether caring is an attribute that is necessarily given to women. Ungerson (1987) describes how many women feel isolated, exploited and manipulated. Lewis and Meredith (1988) portray vividly the daily realities of daughters caring for their sick or disabled mothers. Such research ties in with similar findings about women's work as mothers caring for children with disabilities, particularly in the impact on patterns of daily life, on the isolation of the central carer and difficulties with services, if any. There is less in the literature about women's experiences of caring for people with mental health problems (see Parker, G. 1990; Twigg *et al.*, 1990), except in the area of dementia. As Perring *et al.* (1990) report, the research that exists often compounds gender and kin. The studies they note are also fairly broad and many are difficult to translate into a UK context.

Broadly speaking, then, at a macro-level the variable of gender is important in informal care, since welfare services and the economy depend, as they always have done, on unpaid domestic labour, in particular to support sick and disabled family members. At the mezzo-level, services too have concentrated either on those with no family members or on people whose systems of family support have broken down. The presence of an available female family member clearly alters professionals' perceptions of priority and need. Finally, there are at the micro-level important issues about women's perceptions of themselves, of their roles within families and of their senses of obligation. Qureshi and Walker (1989: 271) write of the 'normative designation' of women as carers and the 'moral imperative' on them to care. This usefully points to the relationship between subjective and objective views of women as carers and underlines the importance of what women say about their experiences and feelings.

Dalley (1993) takes the debate about gender forward by developing a critique of models of care which, based on ideal family types, are individualistic or centred around families. She argues that these are counter to women's interests but also men's, as they stress independence, privacy and market competition: 'Sadly, the admirable impulses that individuals have in caring for their dependents are turned in on themselves rather than being subsumed into a wider ethos of social responsibility across society' (ibid.: p. 124). Women's compulsory altruism is therefore potentially damaging to themselves and it may disregard the perspectives of those who receive their support as compulsory dependents.

Male carers

In this context, the discovery of male carers adds a new dimension to the family-based model of informal care. As we have seen, the traditional interpretation of caring was as women's work, fuelled by studies, personal accounts and pressure group activity in both the UK and the USA. Analysis of GHS data (Green, 1988) and later by Arber and Gilbert (1989) showed that older men contribute significantly to the care of their spouses. Although middle-aged men (under 45, 8 per cent; 45–65 years, 13 per cent) play a significantly lesser role than women of the same age (16 and 28 per cent, respectively, as percentage distribution of total hours of informal care to older people: Arber and Ginn, 1991: 135, see table 8.3), 'older men in co-resident situations break the "normal" gender boundaries of caring' (ibid.: p. 136).

Such research challenges the notion that older people are a 'burden' on younger generations, since it is clear that they are frequently caregivers. It also refutes ideas that men's care is somehow less arduous or competent than that given by women. Arber and Gilbert (1989) did not find men received more support. Issues from this debate are various, particularly the role of marriage and the rewards for both sexes of undertaking caring work. Currently we now accept that caring is not entirely women's work but we are far from equality of labour and responsibility. The focus on male carers has been useful in stressing the importance of the context of relationships as well as challenging stereotypes (see Morris, 1993).

Spouse care

Although the discovery of male carers has been restricted to care in old age, as part of the group of spouse carers the themes can be developed across age groups. Parker (1993) looked at the views of younger people who became disabled after marriage and found it is their partners who provide the majority of care.

Parker talks of the invisibility of marriage in discussions of community care. A focus on spouse care is important for several reasons. First, because it draws attention to both sides of the caring relationship and the dynamics that exist within this and in relationships with others. Second, because it necessitates consideration of people and their relationship in historical terms, factors that superficial assessments neglect. Third, spouse care is evidently not simply a matter of physical labour – there are dimensions of being a couple, perhaps parents, friends and lovers, which challenge the one-dimensional view of people as simply carers or solely as disabled or sick people.

Any discussion of marriage must, of course, acknowledge the growth in the numbers of divorces in the UK. This affects informal care in potentially three ways. First, as McGlone (1992) argues, divorce may become an important factor in reducing the supply of spouse carers. He predicts a rise in the numbers of divorced people from 1 : 31 women aged 65+ and 1 : 34 men of that age group in 1989, to 1 : 7 women and men by the year 2019. Second, divorce may reduce the numbers of daughters-in-law who are willing to care for their partners' parents. We need to be somewhat guarded about this, as Finch and Mason (1993) note that such relationships may continue if there has been substantial assistance in the past. Third, divorce can disrupt those family balances where the income of a male breadwinner can subsidize the care of the female spouse who acts as principal carer in relation to their disabled adult children, his or her parents, or as a volunteer. Such roles may not be so easily adopted if the financial transfer and pooling are substantially altered.

Similarities and differences – carers and age

Our increasing knowledge about the circumstances of carers has focused on age as a key variable. In this section, we explore some of the literature that explains why this should be so. We have chosen to concentrate on older people and young children as carers. We note that there are many important interconnections with other variables, particularly as both of these groups of carers tend to live with the disabled or sick person in the context of a long-standing relationship.

Older carers

One key point from the GHS was its emphasis on older carers, challenging the perennial stereotype of a carer being a middle-aged woman looking after her parents/in-laws. Foremost among older carers are those who care for their spouses and siblings, but as Wenger (1992: 216) points out, increasing numbers of adult children caring for their parents are of retirement age: more than one-third of people are likely to become carers after retirement.

Many older people who are carers would count as being heavily involved, and co-residence is often a characteristic. Wenger writes: 'Elderly carers are therefore engaged in demanding, time-consuming and emotionally draining terminal care' (ibid.: p. 209). Many carers looking after their spouse receive little help, but they perceive their role to have rewards. For example, Pollitt *et al.* (1991) note that the key difference between older spouses and other carers is the way they perceive their partners and their insistence on independence, which reflects the couple's frequent interdependence.

There would appear to be significant points of difference between older carers and carers from other age groups; however, it is difficult to disentangle them from long-term or marital relationships, from the living-together status, from the terminal illness of many recipients and the degree of physical ill-health of the carer. In terms of service provision, these points need to be recognized. This may mean developing services that maintain relationships, are home-centred, that help both parties and are sensitive to fluctuating needs. The literature surrounding carers of people with dementia is particularly helpful in illustrating what is useful, relevant and appropriate (Levin *et al.*, 1989).

An important subset of older carers, where their ageing is also important, is that of older people caring for children who are handicapped or have long-term health problems. Grant (1990) has explored the circumstances of parents with adult children who have learning disabilities and Wright and Alison (1991) have looked broadly at parents whose adult children have cerebral palsy. In his study of older carers from North Wales, Grant (1986: 350) observed that such carers are frequently poor and isolated:

> The stresses as well as the rewards of caring for mentally handicapped adults were not difficult to identify. There were anxieties about the future stemming from anticipated deterioration in the health or mobility of the carer, the lack of statutory services, the desire to avoid obligating relatives or friends or neighbours to assume responsibility for care and, in short, the inability to control what the outcome might be.

Such findings confirm work with families who support relatives with a long-term mental health problem (e.g. Pilling, 1991). Clearly, a much greater understanding is required of the needs of carers who have taken on responsibilities for decades and see them as life-long. Many such carers will have had little if any relationship with service providers and many will have coped with sizeable difficulties single-handed. Their own disabilities or poor health may be the factor that brings them to services' attention at the very time when they are least able to articulate their needs or views.

Children as carers

Parker's (1992: 16) observation that 'over the past few years, this issue has generated much heat but relatively little light', is crucial to bear in mind when discussing the subject of children who provide long-term physical or personal care for family members. One research project which did raise this issue was part of the Department of Health's initiative on *Demonstration Districts for Informal Carers, 1986–1989.* Hills (1991) notes that a survey of teachers in secondary schools in Sandwell found they knew of 169 secondary school age (11+) children who were carers. Around half were under fourteen years of age and the teachers felt a third of them were underachieving at school (Hills, 1991: 11).

Interestingly, research focused on parents who are disabled suggests that they are keen to avoid involving their children in caring tasks (Parker, 1993). The literature reflecting the views of disabled mothers also makes it clear that most are very sensitive to the amount of care given by their children and its appropriateness (Lonsdale, 1990).

Life after caring

In the case of dementia, we have some evidence that ceasing to be a carer – on the death or move to a residential facility of the person affected – can relieve stress and improve well-being (Levin *et al.*, 1989). As one might expect, then, the experience of stopping to be a carer is varied. We have little information about its effects when other conditions are involved, nor how it affects people in the long term. Does the experience of acting as a carer significantly alter people's perceptions and lifestyles? Importantly, does giving care affect one's position as an eventual recipient? Parker (1993: 122) notes that some carers in her study felt more independent and self-reliant, although this might extend to feeling 'separate' from their contemporaries.

Similarities and differences – the experience of black carers

The White Paper *Caring for People* (Department of Health, 1989) made brief reference to the needs of people from black and ethnic minority communities:

> The Government recognises that people from different cultural backgrounds may have particular care needs and problems. Minority communities may have different concepts of community care and it is important that service providers are sensitive to these variations. Good community care will take account of the circumstances of minority communities and will be planned in consultation with them.
>
> (Department of Health, 1989: para. 2.9)

It may be useful to try and unpick some of the ideas behind this quote.

Three main points arise from the literature. First, the similarity of carers' experiences in terms of their frequent isolation, neglect and complex patterns of physical and emotional variables. Second, despite this, race factors are important and pervasive in the relationship of carers to services, in the relationship between carers and the person being cared for, and in relation to the wider sociopolitical environment of contemporary Britain. In terms of services, Atkin and Rollings (1992) summarize some of the research which identifies barriers to the receipt of relevant services. It is not simply a matter of imparting information; they note that underused and inappropriate services are governed by providers' ethnocentric assumptions. They insist that: 'Accessibility, acceptability and negotiation, as well as impact of provision need to be considered by services' (ibid.: p. 415).

Third, the experience of black carers and carers from other ethnic minorities needs to be considered in relation to particular demographic trends (see Williams, 1990). Briefly, these include the rising numbers of elderly people from minority groups as the age distribution of black groups begins to resemble that of the white majority. There is also the factor of geography, in that ethnic minorities may live in supportive if deprived communities, but some live in isolation from other meaningful networks. Importantly, there is also a wide variation in the family structure of ethnic minority groups. For example, Atkin and Rollings (1992: 409) point out that among the Asian population, family organization may be 'bi-modal'; that is, some people living in extended family groupings while others may live alone.

As yet, we have little information about the impact of race on disabilities and patterns of sickness. It has proved difficult to disentangle the factors concerning race, immigration, income, discrimination and beliefs about illness and health. For example, mental ill-health in old age may be affected by early trauma, loss and lack of supportive networks, and so may affect some minority groups disproportionally. However, the over-representation of younger black people in residential mental health services has often been ascribed to factors emphasizing social control (Ahmad, 1990). We have only recently begun to analyse carers' experiences in such contexts. Baxter *et al.* (1990) offer useful insights into the position of parents whose children are undergoing assessment; they will be clearly relevant to future assessments in community care.

Neighbours and friends

Although the much-quoted definition of community care from the DHSS White Paper *Growing Older* (DHSS, 1981) links together family, neighbours and friends in one web of community care, studies show that there are great differences between these groups of carers.

Abrams *et al.* (1989) make the point that we need to have a proper understanding of how neighbours normally relate to each other in contemporary Britain. They see it as a 'managed relationship', in which people make deliberate decisions about their time and energies and generally prefer and expect neighbours to be distant, casual and guarded. They anticipate help in emergencies and a certain degree of pleasant behaviour. In most circumstances, people hope to be able to reciprocate help, which is generally confined to practical matters. Previously more intensive patterns of neighbourliness were generally a conscious reaction to difficult social contexts, such as dangerous work environments, geographical isolation, deprivation and insecurity. Abrams *et al.* (1989) question whether we would want such social conditions, which seem to compel 'neighbourliness'.

Nonetheless, within this general context there are many individuals and groups for whom neighbours are important at certain times of their lives. It is, perhaps, after the birth of children, or retirement, or unemployment, that the neighbourhood and neighbours become more central to people's lives. In the context of community care, however, it is important to distinguish between organized neighbourhood care, a local voluntary group and the organized neighbour. Terming each the informal sector of care is not particularly helpful or accurate, let alone conflating it with the commercial sector.

The organized neighbour

This category of informal care is one which has been given prominence by the Kent Community Care pilot models of case management. In essence, a neighbour (that includes a person living locally as well as in proximity) undertakes, by agreement with the person concerned and the professional who is coordinating care, a number of tasks for which he or she is rewarded by token or low payment. The term 'quasi-volunteer' has been used or the term 'helper'. Challis and Davies (1986) describe how affective relationships developed in their experimental scheme, but that the formal arrangements were also useful in guaranteeing a certain regularity, reliability and quality.

Other voluntary help is given for no financial reward, although there are likely to be invisible benefits for the volunteer. As Leat (1990) points out, voluntary activity has been driven by its potential rather than evidence of its success. It has clear problems in being comprehensive, in that it is unequally represented in certain geographical areas and with certain groups or individuals. It also has a 'haphazard relationship to need' (Leat, 1990: 288). Even more fundamental are the relationships between volunteers and recipients, particularly as more organized voluntary groups move into contractual services for those most in need of services.

Informal care: New models

The emergence of HIV/AIDS has challenged many of our existing no-tions about informal care. Such an often-stigmatizing condition has meant that traditional family structures are not always supportive. As Warren (1990) notes, many people with HIV/AIDS want to live near treatment centres and so are distant from their relatives.

Sometimes in place of relatives and sometimes alongside them, informal care is often provided by partners, friends, volunteers and self-help groups – the membership of each sector being rather fluid and difficult to distin-guish. Warren debates whether such large surrogate extended families exist, because many of the groups within which the disease is transmitted are minorities, which although discriminated against, can draw on the strengths of their collective experiences. She notes that like all informal care networks, they too can be patchy and variable. It would appear, therefore, that we should be equally careful in endowing this form of informal care with ill-conceived notions about its comprehensiveness. It illustrates again the importance of looking at the characteristics of the carer, the relationship of the individuals involved in conjunction with the condition of the person receiving care.

Care provided by relations has its limitations suggests Sinclair (1990). He notes it is:

- variable in terms of relationship and geography;
- not proportional to need;
- not possible to consciously create;
- potentially full of stresses and strains.

Sinclair broadens the debate in terms of providing support and encourag-ing carers by asking what would work. There are many services which appear to be very useful to carers, but we also need to consider items such as tax incentives, leave entitlement, housing allocations and social security provisions. These are under-researched areas.

Costing care

Nolan *et al.* (1990) point out that an important factor in whether or not carers perceive themselves to be stressed is pressure from the financial costs of caring. There are many areas in which care and finance are linked, and in focusing on some elements in relation to carers we must necessarily be selective. In this section, we shall look at the costs of caring, and the debate about whether carers should be financially compensated for their work. Naturally, this is difficult to separate from issues concerning the level of income and resources of the person who receives care. There is evidence to suggest that when either the carer or the disabled person or both have resources, they may be used to build up networks which transfer the hands-on physical tending work to other paid persons (Parker, R. 1990), or be used to pay for telephones, taxis and private therapists to provide support, solve intractable transport difficulties or arrange individual and controllable services. However, as Arber and Ginn (1992) point out, working-class men and women are more likely than middle-class persons to be involved in the 'heavy' end of co-resident care.

The costs of care for carers

At its most obvious level, the costs of being a carer can be assessed by looking at income and in particular income from employment. There are a variety of ways in which a carer's income can be affected:

- having to leave work;
- having to reduce working hours;
- having to forego overtime/promotion;
- failing to rejoin the labour market;
- taking lower-paid/part-time/conveniently located work;
- dipping in and out of the labour market.

It is estimated that carers of dependent adults comprise one in twelve of all full-time workers and one in six part-time workers (Land, 1992); in the case of elderly spouse carers, it is more difficult to quantify. There are also family patterns to consider, as an individual carer may have a supportive partner or may be single or divorced. In cases of families with disabled children, we know that the mother is likely to delay returning to work but that the father may well increase the number of hours he works (Smyth and Robus, 1989), illustrating how some carers' incomes need to be seen within the wider framework of the household. The debate about employment-based income also excludes those people who are in unemployed households, and that small minority where disability was financially compensated for by the courts.

An Office of Population, Census and Survey report regarding disabled adults also noted that carers' employment is substantially affected, again with differences between the sexes (Martin and White, 1988). In particular, when considering married couples, those men with disabled wives appeared to be most negatively affected. As Parker (1993) points out, in her research of twenty-two married couples, this may be the result of several interconnected factors: there are fewer part-time jobs for men, women are less likely to have any employment-based compensation schemes, and women are less likely to have occupational benefits. For almost all couples, however, she identifies a 'lifetime of scrimping and scraping' (ibid.: p. 81).

Much research has concentrated on carers of employment age who are involved in physical and personal support. For those who care for people diagnosed as mentally ill, there is less evidence, although much of the research on carers of older people includes those with dementia. In respect of those with younger partners, MacCarthy (1988) reports that many spouses are unemployed and perhaps unemployable to some extent and have few social contacts. Mental health problems that occur later often result in relatives having to sort out debts which can be 'the focus for much conflict and distress' (ibid.: p. 217).

The effects of caring are naturally individual and often hidden, but regarding employment we are now able to say that 'combining care-giving and paid work is the *rule* rather than the exception' (Glendinning, 1992: 105), though this spans the spectrum from informal helpers to those heavily involved. Employment, therefore, has to be brought into the mainstream of the debate about community care: not only because of its instrumental and intrinsic income generation, but also because it appears to play a significant role in providing emotional release and satisfaction. This shows itself when discussing the role of socially valued tasks, such as work in relation to people with disabilities themselves (Wertheimer, 1992).

One further group of carers are those not in employment and who rely on social security provision for their subsistence. In the UK, this provision has grown from concern about the stereotypical carer (a spinster) who gave up her career to care for ageing parent(s). Invalid Care Allowance (ICA) has been extended to cover married women, but as Glendinning (1988: 136) summarizes, many of the issues discussed in the 1974 White Paper on *Social Security Provision for Chronically Sick and Disabled People* (DHSS, 1974) are still highly relevant. These include:

• Provision for carers with paid employment that takes them over the threshold for claiming ICA.
• The low level of ICA.
• The dependence of carers' benefits on the disability benefits of the person receiving care.
• The exclusion of carers over retirement age from claiming carers' benefits.
• The resultant financial dependence of carers on others in the household, including the person with disabilities.

As we shall see later, this last point is particularly pertinent and appears to cover many people looking after people regardless of the type of disability involved.

Receiving a carer's wage

Whether carers should be paid for the work they do is an issue that raises many questions concerning equity, costs and emotions. As Ungerson (1990) points out, this is a subject which rests very heavily on the economic position of women within the family and within the wider employment market. If informal care were to be costed and paid, she argues that it would become 'prohibitively expensive' and 'all care would be transferred to the formal sector for pure cost reasons' (ibid.: p. 28). Alternatively, more men might be attracted to this area of work or more services might be organized collectively.

Such debates might seem impractical at a time when wages for carers do not appear on the policy agenda, but the issues underlie other related debates. The first is who should receive compensation in respect of the costs of disability or illness? The current benefits system straddles this question by awarding small payments to both parties (carers and the disabled person) in some circumstances. Disabled people, or their advocates, might argue that carers have no automatic right to an income, since there is no guarantee of the standard or quality of the service they provide, nor is there any contract or explicit agreement about commitment or rights. The second issue is that of payment for quasi-volunteers, which is discussed elsewhere in this chapter. Third, there is the issue of age. As we saw earlier, many carers are older people; with respect to the care they give, a carers' wage would have to be a payment for services instead of compensation for loss of employment. If we are to be fair to them, this would have to be accepted; it would also challenge the inherent ageism of the current benefits system.

Naturally, there are many costs of caring other than loss of income, whether in the present or in the future. There is considerable debate as how best to measure and monetize opportunity costs. When a disabled person goes into a residential or nursing home, there are the costs of travel, gifts, extra items for personal use, let alone help with fees which many families provide. We have little knowledge of these costs, but research into the provisions of the NHS and Community Care Act 1990 will undoubtedly bring them into sharper relief. Recent research (Wright, 1992) has indicated that many people already turn to charities for such help.

Empowering carers

The focus upon carers has become both individualistic and problem-centred. In this section, we look briefly at the potential for carers to act collectively and politically. Such an approach again emphasizes that carers are not a homogeneous group – they may have totally different views and care, of course, varies in times of political persuasion, class, income, race, age and gender.

Organized carers may not describe themselves as carers. MENCAP (the Royal Society for Mentally Handicapped Children and Adults), for example, describes itself in terms of its members' common relationship to people with learning disabilities or mental handicap. They are often parents; frequently, however, they are parents of adult children. They may act as a pressure group, as providers of a service, a self-help group or information network. To a great extent, they may, with variations over time and geographical region, act as voluntary organizations (see Harding, 1986).

Such groups of carers now tread a fine line between representing those who are carers and those who act as broader advocates for social change. MENCAP describes how its early role was confrontational: 'One of the main reasons for the success of the parent movement is its insistence in challenging the professional and the established order of things. In the early days it inevitably collided with authorities' (MENCAP, 1986: 8). Strain may always exist within such large groups of carers, some of whom are actively providing substantial physical or personal care, some of whom are removed from that aspect but who remain actively involved as relatives overseeing or augmenting care provision, and some of whom wish involvement with varied input as carers' representatives in service planning and quality assurance.

In the area of dementia, the Alzheimer's Disease Society (ADS) illustrates another issue, that of maintaining a balance between carers and professionals. As a younger organization, there are clear parallels with MENCAP's growth, as the ADS encourages and disseminates medical and social research to its members. Here there is still marked congruence between informal and formal carers, with both sectors keen to raise the profile of the disease and its effects, typically on spouse carers but also on adult children. Many carers in this area face acute difficulties in acting collectively because of the demands of dementia and also because carers are likely to have their own health problems, restricted mobility and lack of support structures. It may be that services need to acknowledge these restrictions and enable carers to meet together not simply for mutual support, but in order to articulate common concerns (Hettiaratchy and Manthorpe, 1992). In both MENCAP and ADS, there is also the problem of managing an organization while maintaining an individualized focus.

The final illustration here is of the National Schizophrenia Fellowship (NSF), whose work includes uncovering government inconsistencies and discrepancies over the closure of long-stay mental hospitals. Such relatives' associations criticize aspects of the closure of long-stay hospitals and draw attention to the risks involved in maintaining people in the community. To some extent, this may be a reaction against the idea that people with mental health problems are not ill and it may also reflect relatives' strong feelings that support is inadequate. Barnham (1992: 132) comments:

> Indeed it is precisely because some relatives have been isolated in their tasks, and the social rights of patients and relatives neglected, that relatives' associations have sometimes been forced into reactive

positions. In such beleaguered and lonely conditions of existence it is scarcely surprising that the National Schizophrenia Fellowship should report that anxious relatives not infrequently resort to the police as the agency seemingly most willing to intervene and the most promising route to the official legitimation of the tribulations that beset them.

The NSF illustrates the tension that may underlie relationships between carers and professionals. Its strengths lie in its ability to articulate the problems of its members who may find its peer-group support invaluable and unique. This results in the NSF having a political impact and political visibility at levels of policy making which are highly influential. A stereotypical view of powerless carers needs to address the very real differences between certain sections.

The future for carers in this area is open to debate. The provisions of the NHS and Community Care Act 1990 may mean a transfer of resources or increased contractual relationships between social services departments and voluntary groups. Groups of organized carers will have to make decisions about their ability to deliver services. They should, at the level of community care planning and health needs assessment planning, be more involved with statutory agencies. Larger groups and those with paid staff will obviously be able to respond to these overtures. It remains to be seen how individual carers' relationships with their representative organizations evolve and how the notions of empowerment work in reality.

The spotlight thrown on carers does obscure the concept that caring itself is socially constructed to some extent. It may not be all carers' choice to provide personal or physical assistance, but there may be no alternative or little acceptable alternative. We know that carers say they would like more services and finance. That they are not willing to use their labour as a bargaining instrument is fortunate for the Treasury; to do so would probably create a moral panic about the dumping of relatives and the demise of family values.

A lack of appropriate housing, inadequate personal care services, an insufficient income and an inaccessible environment force many disabled people into accepting help from their relatives. Choice is restricted for all parties. We should not be surprised that this perversion of relationships is problematic; the challenge for those implementing community care is to empower both carers and those receiving care from whatever quarter.

The other side of the coin

In this chapter, I have outlined how recent government policy has emphasized the quality and quantity of informal carers' work in supporting vulnerable individuals. However, such a view runs the risk of seeing all carers as well-motivated and all relationships as unproblematic. Recent research (combined also with much anecdote) has begun to identify situations where carers fail to protect – or mistreat or neglect – individuals whom they have a degree of power over by nature of their vulnerability. I am deliberately avoiding the term 'are responsible for', as it is misleading and inaccurate. In the area of informal care, abuse and neglect have begun to be recognized as possible dimensions of the caring experience.

Initial interest in the UK was in the area of elder abuse (initially termed 'granny-battering'). However, criticisms of long-stay hospital provision, which we might call 'institutional abuse', have been made across the range of long-stay patients and their conditions. There is still no certainty about the numbers of people affected or at risk and we are reliant on American data, but research is starting. In the meantime, efforts have been directed to analysing possible explanations for abuse or mistreatment (the latter phrase including neglect) and possible helping mechanisms that can reduce the risk, assist victims and alter the behaviour in question.

Phillipson and Biggs (1992: 19) provide a useful summary of the explanations that have been developed in respect of elder abuse within the individualized domestic setting. These include stress on carers, the lack of reciprocity within a relationship, the ways in which identities undergo change and the structured dependency of older people. Such an analysis shows that researchers have moved beyond a simplistic view of mistreatment as being solely the result of intolerable stress on an over-burdened relative. Possible helping mechanisms include procedures and policies for helping reduce risk and offering assistance to the vulnerable person (Manthorpe, 1993). Practical interventions include providing services which separate individuals in the guise of respite, day care or residential options. They may also include counselling or other therapeutic assistance (see Penhale, 1992).

From this initial interest in elder abuse, policy-makers and practitioners have also developed work on identifying mistreatment or abuse among other vulnerable adults. Much initial interest in this area came from the reported case of a young woman, Beverley Lewis, whose death prompted specific and general interest into the powers of intervention when a mentally incapacitated adult may be in need of protection (Law Commission, 1991).

In the area of learning disabilities, the concept of heightened vulnerability of adults and children has been proposed:

> . . . individuals with a mental handicap often have fewer situation safeguards to protect them from sexual exploitation. They frequently lead relatively isolated lives and may be cared for in quite intimate ways by other people.
>
> (Brown and Craft, 1989: 2)

Such an analysis avoids victim-blaming and focuses on preconditions. It has the added feature of not differentiating between informal (family) carers and paid staff; either may be able to exercise inappropriate power when external controls are minimal, when opportunities present themselves, when resistance is low and when internal inhibitions are overridden.

There is the danger that procedures might become over-bureaucratized and that mutual suspicion might come to dominate relationships between carers and service providers. Equally damaging might be the notion that services, being targeted on those at risk, will become stigmatizing as they are directed towards carers who are perceived to be inadequate or possibly dangerous.

Policy and professional responses to carers

In policy terms, carers have moved from being relatively invisible to a position where their needs are being increasingly recognized, if not met. Their invisibility was perhaps due to a combination of factors: carers do not usually define themselves as carers, nor do they form groups or act collectively. In many ways, their role excludes them from public life and is also physically and mentally exhausting. For many, activity on the public stage has often meant involvement in activities organized around the disability or medical condition of the person they look after; itself often a reliable and practical source of information, support and companionship.

Here, though, we concentrate on *policy* and central government policy in particular. It is important to remember that this is not the only policy-making body and that policies, once made, have to be implemented.

Government policy

The Griffiths' Report (1988) acknowledges that families, friends, neighbours and other local people provide most care to people in need. He identifies two tasks for publicly provided services: '. . . to support and where possible strengthen these networks of carers' (para. 3.2) and '. . . to identify where these caring networks have broken down, or cannot meet the needs, and decide what public services are desirable to fill the gap' (para. 3.3).

The notion of support is fundamental and is seen again in the White Paper, *Caring for People* (Department of Health, 1989). However, Griffiths' view of caring networks is less widely accepted. Wenger's (1992) study goes some way in moving the notion of network from metaphor to reality, as her longitudinal research describes a variety of networks, their ability to be supportive deriving from different types of relationships. Clearly, findings such as these, which illustrate that areas with stable populations have more caring capacity, potentially conflicts with other government policies that call for mobility of labour or encourage dispersed housing. *Caring for People* (Department of Health, 1989) translates the Griffiths' Report into policy. One of its six main objectives is 'to ensure that service providers make practical support for carers a high priority' (para. 1.11). It follows this with an analysis of the contributions of carers:

> The majority of carers take on these responsibilities willingly, but the Government recognises that many need help to be able to manage what can become a heavy burden. Their lives can be made much easier if the right support is there at the right time, and a key responsibility of statutory service providers should be to do all they can to assist and support carers. Helping carers to maintain their valuable contribution to the spectrum of care is both right and a sound investment. Help may take the form of providing advice and support as well as practical services such as day, domiciliary and respite care.
>
> (Department of Health, 1989: para. 2.3)

This paragraph is quoted at some length as it encapsulates current government thinking in this area. Carers are deemed to be important, to be willing, to be deserving of help. There are many common threads with previous government documents such as *Better Services for the Mentally Handicapped* (DHSS, 1971), which emphasizes the strain placed on families (p. 3), *A Happier Old Age* (DHSS, 1978), which focuses on the growing demands on relatives but suggests a minority do not choose to provide support (p. 13), and *Growing Older* (DHSS, 1981), which acknowledges community care services assist caring families and points out that the vast majority can and do care (p. 37). Each of these documents throws up points that continue to be relevant; none of course use the word 'carer' until *Caring for People*. The NHS and Community Care Act 1990 itself talks of 'private carers', a significant departure from Griffiths' caring networks.

The service response: Assessing carers' needs

Twigg (1989) identifies three models which seem to explain how services conceptualize their relationship with carers. These are referred to by Alaszewski and McIntosh in this volume. The ambiguities of the relationship between service provider and carer are acknowledged in policy implementation documents: 'In weighing the perceptions of carers, the practitioner must take account of all vested interests and give due weight to each perception' (Social Services Inspectorate, 1991: 58). The term 'vested interests' is interesting here, as it acknowledges that there may be many complex issues, including that of financial resources. What the individual care manager will do with such information is of course the key. It will be here that negotiation, reaching a consensus, finding a 'good enough' package and planning for emergencies and shortfalls will be the process by which the 'practical support' objective of the White Paper is translated into reality.

A key point in the assessment procedures introduced under the NHS and Community Care Act 1990 is the notion that carers and users may hold conflicting views:

> Because the interests of users and carers may not coincide, both parties should be given the opportunity of separate consultation with an assessing practitioner. If necessary, carers should be offered a separate assessment of their own needs.
>
> (Social Services Inspectorate, 1991: para. 30)

To do this sensitively and meaningfully will be a challenge for assessors. In many ways, they will need time to explore not only the practical, day-to-day tasks involved but also to consider the feelings, perhaps ambivalent, of the carer.

Our knowledge of carers is now quite extensive: we know who does what to whom, and we also know much about the experience of caring and what motivates carers or discourages them (Twigg, 1992: 3). The challenge for practitioners is to place this knowledge into the unique context of people's lives and to use it to develop strategies and interventions that are helpful and effective.

Neill (1989) suggests some key questions that assessors should consider when talking to carers. These include the reminder that the next of kin may not be the person(s) most involved practically or emotionally. Neill (1989: 36) warns:

> You need to understand the carer's problems, state of health and point of view, and take any practical steps possible to relieve immediate difficulty. You may also need a cool head, a good memory of the old person's wishes and strong nerves to prevent yourself from being railroaded into irreversible action.

Neill's work is based on the experiences of social workers assessing older people with dementia-related conditions for residential care; however, the underlying principles for talking to carers are transferable to other groups. In particular, the context of care is a factor which stands out as important in assessing both carers' expressed needs and wishes and seeing them in dynamic relationships. Carers' relationships with people they are looking after have immediate but also historic dimensions. They will also have influential relationships with other key individuals. Assessment therefore needs to reflect these variables, noting in particular those factors which are positive and enjoyable, as attention focused on these may give a radical new perspective to the notion of exploring what support is needed, how it should be supplied and when it might or might not be appropriate to renegotiate patterns of care, protection and domestic life.

Issues of quality

The mismatch of carers' needs and welfare services has been the subject of much research and debate. There is an argument regarding quantity in that services only help to a small extent because they are limited in scope, geography, remit and number. For example, Challis *et al.* (1987: 35–6) found that traditional domiciliary services gave carers few benefits in terms of improving their lifestyle, decreasing mental health problems, reducing their levels of stress or altering their expressed feelings of care being a burden. Younger people with disabilities also reported their disquiet with the services on offer. Borsay's (1986) survey notes services were often thoughtless and rigid in design, characterized by daily unpredictability and inability to respond to individual need. Here the presence of carers appears to reduce the help from statutory services, thereby helping them to target their limited assistance on those who live alone.

More recently, the argument has encompassed the issue of quality, noting that some services are unsatisfactory, inappropriate and tokenistic. It may be useful to look at one piece of recent research in this regard. Jane Hubert examined the experience of respite care for profoundly disabled young adults who had behavioural problems. She talked to twenty families about their experience of respite care (Hubert, 1991). They revealed their dissatisfaction with the *physical care* given to young adults, who were left sitting in wheelchairs or left in bed when wet or soiled. Parents were unhappy with the *medical care*, with drugs being over-administered or misused. They were also upset by aspects of the *social care*, in the sense that staff did not relate to individuals and failed to offer stimulation. Most poignantly, Hubert notes that experiences of short-term respite care had been so distressing for her respondents that most of the mothers (the chief carers) said they would prefer their children to die before them:

> I think I'd rather kill him, quite honestly, I'd rather give him an overdose, than see him go in there. They're not even kept clean, they stink – the whole place stinks. They're suffering there because they can't say any different.

Despite this, some existing services are highly relevant to carers and contribute much to their capacity to cope, their perceptions of stress and their quality of life. The home-help service, with all its rigidities, is perceived to be valued and valuable (Levin *et al.*, 1989). Respite care is likewise undergoing many changes, but it is valued by some carers for the relief from responsibility that it offers. Community nursing services, particularly in the area of mental health and behavioural problems, are viewed favourably, albeit with similar problems of access and resources that are common to other mainstream services (Twigg and Atkin, 1993).

The implementation of the NHS and Community Care Act 1990 will challenge the role and provision of mainstream services. Innovations in care for people with learning disabilities and the development of individual programme plans are areas which have already demonstrated that there will be tensions between new models of service delivery and carers' expectations. Leat (1990) identifies several examples of new approaches to carer support: neighbourhood care schemes; sitting schemes; flexible care attendance schemes; home-based flexible respite; and information, advice and support. The key themes to these are that they are designed to be flexible, to be based in or near a person's home, and that they build on what carers have long identified as missing from large-scale remote services, i.e. they should give carers a degree of choice and control. Care management, of course, will be an integral part of accessing such services in terms of information and financial support.

The NHS and Community Care Act 1990 also calls for encouragement of the independent sector in the area of domiciliary care. Few carers have significant relationships with the commercial sector of care other than in residential/nursing home provision on a long-term basis. Research is required to track the ability of carers to negotiate with commercial organizations over domiciliary services and to develop understandings of mutual relationships.

Finally, under the heading of 'quality', it is important to consider the quality of carers' lives and how services may enhance this. As Sinclair (1990) notes in respect of broad issues of community care, much policy discussion ignores the interdependence of many factors. This is clearly so with carers, whose quality of life may be affected by their own personal situation, by factors affecting the recipients of their care, and by complex relationships between the two, the wider family and broader social relationships.

Conclusion

The NHS and Community Care Act 1990 holds out great hopes for carers. In this chapter, we have seen that carers are no more a homogeneous group than people whose disability or sickness means they rely on other people for assistance in day-to-day living. The literature and research has moved from simplistic and elusive categorizing to an analysis of complex interactions and transactions between individuals. In the next decade, it will be interesting to note if carers are supported and empowered by the new system of social care or whether they remain marginalized as the territory of welfare is fought over by the statutory and independent sectors.

References

Abrams, P., Abrams, S., Humphrey, R. and Snaith, R. (1989). *Neighbourhood Care and Social Policy.* London: HMSO.

Ahmad, B. (1990). *Black Perspectives in Social Work.* Birmingham: Venture Press.

Arber, S. and Gilbert, N. (1989). Men: The forgotten carers. *Sociology, 23*(1): 111–18.

Arber, S. and Ginn, J. (1991). *Gender and Later Life.* London: Sage.

Arber, S. and Ginn, J. (1992). Class and caring: A forgotten dimension. *Sociology, 26*(4): 619–34.

Atkin, K. and Rollings, J. (1992). Informal care in Asian and Afro/Caribbean communities: A literature review. *British Journal of Social Work, 22*(4): 405–418.

Barnham, P. (1992). *Closing the Asylum: The Mental Patient in Modern Society.* Harmondsworth: Penguin.

Baxter, C., Ward, L., Poonia, K. and Naidirshaw, Z. (1990). *Double Discrimination.* London: King's Fund/Commission for Racial Equality.

Biggs, A. and Oliver, J. (eds) (1985). *Caring: Experiences of Looking After Disabled Relatives.* London: Routledge and Kegan Paul.

Borsay, A. (1986). *Disabled People in the Community.* London: Bedford Square Press.

Brown, H. and Craft, A. (eds) (1989). *Thinking the Unthinkable: Papers on Sexual Abuse and People with Learning Difficulties.* London: Family Planning Association Training Unit.

Brown, H. and Smith, H. (eds) (1992). *Normalisation: A Reader for the Nineties.* London: Routledge.

Challis, D. and Davies, B. (1986). *Case Management in Community Care.* Aldershot: Gower.

Challis, D., Chessum, R., Chesterman, J., Luckett, R. and Woods, B. (1987). *Community care for the frail elderly: An urban experiment. British Journal of Social Work, 18:* 13–42 (suppl.).

Dalley, G. (1993). Caring: A legitimate interest of older women. In Bernard, M. and Meade, K. (eds), *Women Come of Age.* London: Edward Arnold.

Department of Health (1989). *Caring for People: Community Care in the Next Decade and Beyond.* Cm. 849. London: HMSO.

Department of Health and Social Security (1971). *Better Services for the Mentally Handicapped.* Cmnd 4683. London: HMSO.

Department of Health and Social Security (1974). *Social Security Provision for Chronically Sick and Disabled People.* London: HMSO.

Department of Health and Social Security (1978). *A Happier Old Age.* London: HMSO.

Department of Health and Social Security (1981). *Growing Older.* Cmnd 8173. London: HMSO.

Finch, J. and Mason, J. (1993). *Negotiating Family Responsibilities.* London: Routledge.

Glendinning, C. (1988). Dependency and interdependency: The incomes of informal carers and the impact of social security. In Baldwin, S., Parker, G. and Walker, R. (eds), *Social Security and Community Care.* Aldershot: Avebury.

Glendinning, C. (1992). Employment and 'community care': Policies for the 1990s. *Work, Employment and Society*, 6(1): 103–111.

Grant, G. (1986). Older carers, interdependence and the care of mentally handicapped adults. *Ageing and Society*, 6(3): 333–53.

Grant, G. (1990). Elderly parents and handicapped children: Anticipating the future. *Journal of Ageing Studies*, 4(4): 359–74.

Green, H. (1988). *Informal Carers*. London: HMSO.

Griffiths, R. (1988). *Community Care: Agenda for Action*. London: HMSO.

Harding, T. (1986). *A Stake in Planning: Joint Planning and the Voluntary Sector*. London: National Council of Voluntary Organisations.

Hettiaratchy, P. and Manthorpe, J. (1992). A carers' group for families of patients with dementia. In Jones, G. and Miesen, B. (eds), *Care – Giving in Dementia*. London: Routledge.

Hills, D. (1991). *Carer Support in the Community: Evaluation of the Department of Health Initiative: 'Demonstration Districts for Informal Carers' 1986–1989*. Department of Health/Social Services Inspectorate. London: HMSO.

Hubert, J. (1991). *No Place Like Home? Crisis in the Care of Young Adults with Severe Learning Difficulties: A Study of 20 Families*. London: King's Fund.

Land, H. (1991). Time to care. In MacLean, M. and Groves, D. (eds), *Women's Issues in Social Policy*. London: Routledge.

Land, H. (1992). A damaging dichotomy: Women and part-time v full-time employment. *Benefits*, September/October, pp. 10–13.

Law Commission (1991). *Mentally Incapacitated Adults and Decision-Making: An Overview*. Consultation Paper No. 119. London: HMSO.

Leat, D. (1990). Overwhelming voluntary failure: Strategies for change. In Sinclair, I., Parker, R., Leat, D. and Williams, J. (eds), *The Kaleidoscope of Care*. London: HMSO.

Levin, E., Sinclair, I. and Gorbach, P. (1989). *Families, Services and Confusion in Old Age*. Aldershot: Gower.

Lewis, J. and Meredith, B. (1988). *Daughters Who Care*. London: Routledge.

Lonsdale, S. (1990). *Women and Disability*. London: Macmillan.

MacCarthy, B. (1988). The role of relatives. In Lavender, A. and Holloway, F. (eds), *Community Care in Practice: Services for the Continuing Care Client*. Chichester: Wiley.

Manthorpe, J. (1993). Elder abuse and key areas in social work. In Decalmer, P. and Glendenning, F. (eds), *The Mistreatment of Elderly People*. London: Sage.

Martin, J. and White, A. (1988). *The Financial Circumstances of Disabled Adults Living in Private Households*. London: HMSO.

McGlone, F. (1992). *Disability and Dependency in Old Age: A Demographic and Social Audit*. London: Family Policy Studies Centre.

MENCAP (1986). *Day Services Today and Tomorrow*. London: MENCAP.

Morris, J. (1993). *Independent Lives: Community Care and Disabled People*. London: Macmillan.

Neill, J. (1989). *Assessing Elderly People for Residential Care: A Practical Guide*. London: National Institute for Social Work Research Unit.

Nolan, M., Grant, G. and Ellis, N. (1990). Stress is in the eye of the beholder: Reconceptualising the measurement of carer burden. *Journal of Advanced Nursing*, 15(5): 544–55.

Parker, G. (1990). *With Due Care and Attention*, 2nd edn. London: Family Policy Studies Centre.

Parker, G. (1992). Counting care: Numbers and types of informal carers. In Twigg, J. (ed.), *Carers: Research and Practice*. London: HMSO.

Parker, G. (1993). *With This Body: Caring and Disability in Marriage*. Buckingham: Open University Press.

Parker, R. (1990). Private domestic help and care. In Sinclair, I., Parker, R., Leat, D. and Williams, J. (eds), *The Kaleidoscope of Care*. London: HMSO.

Penhale, B. (1992). Elder abuse: An overview. *Elders*, *1*(3): 36–48.

Perring, C., Twigg, J. and Atkin, K. (1990). *Families Caring for People Diagnosed as Mentally Ill: The Literature Re-examined*. London: HMSO.

Phillipson, C. and Biggs, S. (1992). *Understanding Elder Abuse: A Training Manual for Helping Professionals*. Harlow: Longman.

Pilling, S. (1991). *Rehabilitation and Community Care*. London: Routledge.

Pollitt, P., Anderson, I. and O'Connor, D. (1991). For better or for worse: The experience of caring for an early dementing spouse. *Ageing and Society*, *11*(4): 443–70.

Qureshi, H. and Walker, A. (1989). *The Caring Relationship: Elderly People and Their Families*. London: Macmillan.

Sinclair, I. (1990). Carers: Their contribution and quality of life. In Sinclair, I., Parker, R., Leat, D. and Williams, J. (eds), *The Kaleidoscope of Care*. London: HMSO.

Smyth, M. and Robus, N. (1989). *The Financial Circumstances of Families with Disabled Children Living in Private Households*. London: HMSO.

Social Services Inspectorate (1991). *Care Management and Assessment: Practitioners' Guide*. London: HMSO.

Twigg, J. (1989). Models of carers: How do social care agencies conceptualise their relationship with informal carers? *Journal of Social Policy*, *18*(1): 53–66.

Twigg, J. (ed.) (1992). *Carers: Research and Practice*. London: HMSO.

Twigg, J. and Atkin, K. (1993). *Carers Perceived*. Buckingham: Open University Press.

Twigg, J., Atkin, K. and Perring, C. (1990). *Carers and Services: A Review of Research*. London: HMSO.

Ungerson, C. (1987). *Policy is Personal, Sex, Gender and Informal Care*. London: Tavistock.

Ungerson, C. (ed.) (1990). *Gender and Caring: Work and Welfare in Britain and Scandinavia*. Brighton: Harvester-Wheatsheaf.

Warren, P. (1990). *New Perspectives on Informal Networks – HIV Infection/AIDS*. Bulletin No. 7. Canterbury: Personal Social Services Research Unit, University of Kent.

Wenger, G.C. (1992). *Help in Old Age – Facing up to Change*. Liverpool: Liverpool University Press.

Wertheimer, A. (1992). Give us the tools. *Community Care*, 6 February, pp. 16–17.

Williams, J. (1990). Elders from black and minority ethnic communities. In Sinclair, I., Parker, R., Leat, D. and Williams, J. (eds), *The Kaleidoscope of Care*. London: HMSO.

Wright, F. (1992). *Fee Shortfalls in Residential and Nursing Homes: The Impact on the Voluntary Sector*. London: Age Concern Institute of Gerontology.

Wright, F. and Alison, V. (1991). *Still Caring*. London: The Spastics Society.

7 Measuring service quality

Michael Beazley

Introduction

Developments stemming from the NHS and Community Care Act 1990 have renewed debate about improving the quality of care in the community, and the means by which standards can be most effectively guaranteed within a new framework of 'enabling' policy for local government. The language and ideas of present-day quality policy borrow heavily from the business world, first tested in the National Health Service (NHS) in the form of a managed internal market, and now tentatively introduced to the world of personal social services (PSS). It would be difficult not to be in favour of quality, but the criteria of quality and the most valid ways of measuring them appear to be seen differently through the eyes of policy makers, service workers and service users.

In this chapter, I shall look at some of the tensions between ideas about improving quality and consider some of the relevant content of policy and legislation for community care.

Quality and the purchasing role

In social services departments' (SSDs) future and evolving role as purchasers, rather than as the main providers of services, the process of quality assurance, including its inspection component, will become even more important. As new purchasing power for social care begins to transfer from the Department of Social Security to local authorities in 1993, the latter will have to develop their quality assurance capacity simultaneously in two directions: first, by 'building in' quality arrangements in delivering and managing services as providers; second, by developing means of ensuring satisfactory standards from independent sector providers, as purchasers of services. Success in both implies a close and influential relationship with providers, supported by a clear contractual agreement which includes quality specifications for services as well as agreement about prices. It also entails agreement about monitoring and inspection arrangements.

An important change in policy represented by this move to an enabling or purchasing role, is in the means by which it is now considered most effective to ensure service quality. The traditional reliance on incremental legislation, policy guidance and other means of central bureaucratic control, is now seen as less important than the management of contractual relationships between social services purchasers and a more diverse range of providers who will supply a growing proportion of the required services. Effectively, the policy devolves further quality responsibility from central to local government, and focuses the role of central government more on controlling and targeting the resources in support of fewer but more specific objectives, and monitoring the results.

Quality issues in community care

Quality is a difficult concept. A growing volume of literature is now available to tell us how to assure it, how to control it, how to inspect it and how to measure it. Ideas about quality in community care now come with the wrappings of a new technical vocabulary of systems, models, indicators and measurements, which might lead some to assume they had stumbled into a world of exact science. Here, given the technical know-how, variables can be readily controlled and services delivered at a standard to satisfy the varied demands of informed customers, who know what they want and can make choices in a marketplace where there is a range of products which compete on criteria of fitness-for-purpose, quality and cost.

So runs the idea of consumer sovereignty, drawn from the experience of quality management in a global product-market and applied to an emerging market approach in the management of community care. Surely, the argument runs, no apology is needed for borrowing from this aspect of manufacturing management theory, from which some industrialized countries may be said to have achieved a powerful economic status? And if quality assurance works to make better cars, washing machines and hi-fi's for a given price, it must have something to contribute to the management of a multi-billion pound service industry called community care?

The application of quality assurance ideas to community care is at an early stage and requires careful translation when transferred to a highly people-intensive service whose objectives are concerned with the state's intervention to relieve the effects of personal and socioeconomic disadvantage, disability, and the breakdown of family and community networks. Some might see only paradox and irony in using the very science of the market, whose dynamics they will see as a main cause of need for personal social services, to manage the operation of services to relieve those needs themselves. For others, pragmatism and practicality will persuade that there is much still to be learned about the most effective ways of running public services to good standards for a reasonable cost: they will accept that some principles of organization and management may be of equal relevance to manufacturing and service industries alike, and can be seen and used in an ideologically neutral way; and that the user of the service can only benefit from an initiative to improve and maintain the quality of care. Some managers will be motivated by the pursuit of quality as a personal ambition, and others persuaded that services users can be more empowered to improve the quality of services if, as the market develops, they are increasingly able to choose from a variety of providers. Those who can provide and maintain better quality services to meet a need for a given cost will succeed because consumers will choose their services in preference to others.

Policy on quality management

In reforming community care policy for the 1990s, government advice to local authorities included guidance on ways of maintaining or improving quality, mainly in the context of the latter's growing role as a purchaser of services from the independent sector. Department of Health practice guidelines (DoH/SSI, 1991) used several key terms to describe techniques and processes likely to help in producing quality services. The umbrella term 'quality assurance' is used to describe 'processes which aim to ensure that concern for quality is built in to services'. These include the production of public statements about intended service standards, and a systematic process to ensure their achievement. 'Quality control' is seen as a component of quality assurance, and describes the processes of checking that quality of the delivered service is being maintained through inspection, monitoring and regular use of objective feedback information. The term 'total quality management' describes an approach in which people at all levels of the workforce are encouraged to take an active responsibility in creating and maintaining a culture of quality in all activities.

The new language of quality is in some danger of being the new bottle for old wine, but essentially points to the need for public commitment to quality by the responsible authorities; planning and managing services to an explicit set of standards; gaining the active commitment of the workforce to those standards; checking regularly to make sure that the service delivered is up to the mark; and then managing changes that may be needed to rectify poor standards.

To those critics seeking a panacea for the inadequacies of community care, it is important to note the limitations of quality assurance ideas and techniques, which cannot themselves be expected to make much impact on the availability or quantity of care. The process of rationing or targeting services involves some of the most difficult local authority decisions in balancing the equation of quality with quantity. Is it wiser to spread resources thinly to provide a just-adequate level of service quality to a hundred people, or improve the quality for a smaller number? This is not to say that quality and quantity are always in such a direct relationship, but that the value of quality assurance practices mainly begins after the point of political/managerial decision about what standards are to be pursued, and the availability of resources has an obvious relevance in fixing the quality 'ceiling'. To this extent, judgement about quality standards cannot be strongly led by the service users, as they often have little or no power to determine the level of resources available to them as individuals, and as yet little knowledge of or choice in the range of services available.

This said, policy reforms strongly emphasize the value of personal choice, and include new statutory rights to choice – initially, in residential care – for a given cost fixed by a local authority. The participation of service users in the community care planning process is also encouraged, and provides a means for SSDs to listen to and take into account users' views.

Criteria of quality

British Standard BS5750 defines quality as 'the totality of features and characteristics of product or services that bear on its ability to satisfy a given need'. It is this definition (and its more recent accompanying notes of interpretation) that appears to be most widely used by SSDs as a starting point in quality development work. It is important to note that in the context of community care, 'needs' have a formal meaning which is contained within a handful of Acts of Parliament, dating onward from the National Assistance Act 1948. Legal definitions of needs are fairly narrow, and mainly refer to needs for particular services (e.g. residential care, home help services), rather than the wider view of needs for social care based on ideas about the quality of life. The ability of a service to 'satisfy' a need is difficult to assess, as there are few examples of studies or effective systems yet in operation which draw directly on the opinions of service users. Instead, an agency is more likely to set out statements of values, philosophy and principles, which it considers will result in a satisfactory service quality if applied in practice. But translating these quality intentions into concrete results, and demonstrating achievements, remains a common difficulty, as both public and professional expectations usually exceed the agency's capacity to resource or manage the necessary change or innovation; nor are there many well-tried and tested measures of user satisfaction with the end-product or outcome.

For the moment, accreditation to the British Standard is heavily based on the existence of quality assurance mechanisms in the providers' management arrangements, and gives little emphasis to the need for direct measures of service outcome or user satisfaction. In contrast to the mechanistic or systems criteria used in the British Standard, other definitions are offered which stress the quality of the overall service to the population, rather than the individual. From a related view of quality in health care, Maxwell (1984) proposes six critical characteristics:

- access to services;
- relevance to need for the whole community;
- equity or fairness in provision for different groups of people;
- effectiveness for individual patients;
- efficiency and economy;
- acceptability to both consumers and providers.

For the Social Services Inspectorate, in its continuing series of published standards, dimensions of quality in residential care are under three broad criteria: quality of care, quality of the environment and the quality of management.

More recently, the Department of Health (1992) surveyed the common themes emerging from work across a sample of SSDs. Their experience in considering definitions suggested that 'the primary definition of Quality should be that of the service user not the service provider or commissioner'. In practice, it emerged that this perspective was often displaced by performance criteria such as value for money, or the capacity to meet management objectives. In other words, the quality of the means, rather than the ends, was used as the main criterion of quality.

Quality outcomes for the service user

Clearly, quality is a highly subjective concept, and in a poorly developed market of providers – where many service users have little direct purchasing power and who are possibly disabled or otherwise disadvantaged – the purchasers (namely central and local government) remain the key actors in determining which needs are to be met, at what quality and at what cost. This is seen by some as an initial step towards a position where, through greater user participation in decision-making, and a greater diversity of service providers, the users' views of quality can ultimately be reflected in their own choice of services.

A less romantic perception would be that community care services usually intervene at a point of personal or family crisis – or just before with a little luck. In these circumstances, the immediate issues about care services may be more about how to get by until tomorrow or next week than they are concerned with 'shopping' for care packages in a quasi-market. Faced with the loss of a partner, the loss of one's home, the loss of liberty as a result of psychotic illness, or immobility from a stroke, social services' users will often depend on care workers to guide them through the possible options, and trust to them that the service received will be of adequate or better quality.

A problem with the language of managerialism is that the meaning of quality has unrealistic overtones of purchasing power and excellence. There is little consonance between the optimism of the new 'managerialism' in pursuit of quality during the 1980s, and the starker realities of entering residential care in old age, following a means test, in the early 1990s.

Viewed more positively, the initiative to manage for quality can be pitched at an obviously useful level; for example, in making sure that a service is regularly evaluated; organizing regular supervision in, and improvement of, the skills of the workforce; or in making sure that service users get reliable and sufficient information when they need to make difficult life decisions. Many basic quality safeguards may be implemented within normal levels of resources and capabilities and are widely accepted as important ingredients of good standards. They are indirect measures of outcome, however, and do not themselves demonstrate a satisfactory service outcome for the user. To date, quality criteria have mainly been concerned with the quality of inputs (e.g. trained staff) or with the qualities of the processes (e.g. the existence of inspection arrangements).

So far as quality of outcome is concerned, it may be the quality of the immediate social and physical environment that is most important for those who live in their own homes. This may be as basic as safety, nutrition and health where, for example, a single person without savings becomes disabled in old age in a house that needs repairs to a leaky roof. For that person, who wishes to stay put at any cost if possible, the quality of community care may be measured by its capacity to fix the roof, get the fire lit and deliver a hot meal three days a week. Finding out what really matters is a basic skill of good assessment and care management, but it is also accessible by other means (e.g. by survey or systematic listening by the organization). When such information is used to inform quality decisions, they are likely to have a ring of authenticity.

Quality aspects of PSS policy

Children's services

The detailed planning of both the Children Act 1989 and the NHS and Community Care Act 1990, provided an opportunity to revise both the content of policy on service quality, as expressed in national guidance on standards, and also the processes by which these standards could be best ensured. Although both Acts – and their voluminous quantities of policy guidance and regulations – are commonly concerned with improving the quality of care, they differ widely in the overall style and method for achieving those ends. For children's services, prescriptive standards were produced in the form of traditional and detailed government regulations, focused almost exclusively on the sharp end of the service. These standards ranged from the detail of how many toilets should be provided in a day nursery, through to the provision of guardians *ad litem* to represent children's own interests in legal proceedings, to the requirement for pay-phones in children's residential homes. The more fundamental purposes of the Children Act 1989 – to redefine and modify the nature and balance of parental responsibilities between the private individual and the state, *in loco parentis* – spawned a major revision of hitherto piecemeal and patchy standards covering almost the full range of children's services.

The legislation and its policy guidance was concerned almost exclusively with the qualities and characteristics of the front-line service. A series of Commencement Orders were used to stagger the implementation time-table of various sections of the legislation. The expectation was that local authorities would absorb the new standards, and manage their own pro-grammes of change to meet them. The policy initiative was concerned primarily with the 'what' rather than the 'how' of improving service quality. Little new guidance was offered about the way in which a public service should organize and train to orientate itself towards a process of quality management, although new standards were pitched at a level clearly in excess of (then) present practice.

A few exceptions to this general statement should be noted, however. The legislation introduced a modest local service planning requirement, a means for dealing with representations and complaints; and through extending the right of children to separate legal representation, gave some acknowledgement to the view that quality is in the eye of the beholder, and not a matter only for professional judgement. Overall, however, the policy changes for children's services did not seek to reflect the new managerialism of the 1980s in their approach to managing quality. Instead, reliance was placed on extending the more traditional central government machinery – that of detailed prescription of the delivered service, and of increasing the range and volume of inspection.

To the extent that the Children Act 1989 reflected a drive for better service quality, it did not address the issues of creating a new management or financial framework. Planning quality improvement in a public service sometimes suffers from the particular uncertainty of one-year-at-a-time financial planning, in a way that would prevent a similarly large independent organization from mounting such an initiative at all. A company going 'up market' with its products or creating new ones may plan its borrowing over many years, in flexible agreement with lenders and on the strength of anticipated achievement and performance within a given period, to offer a worthwhile return on that investment.

One policy problem for the PSS is that such initiatives are vulnerable to the general performance of the economy, and to the resulting annual decisions about the finances made available for public expenditure. The effect of these decisions – first expressed as cash totals for local authority annual expenditure, and second divided between the spending depart-ments of those local authorities – is to guarantee financial uncertainty and complicate the production of a strategy. Neither are the quality outcomes of value of the investment always easy to predict or quantify, as some may only be evident in indirect ways (e.g. the reduction in numbers of chil-dren subject to care orders), which cannot themselves tell the observer whether or not children's quality of life has benefited or not.

Adult services

By way of contrast, the 'quality' content of the NHS and Community Care Act 1990 owes more to the thinking of the business world than it does to the conventional bureaucratic management of policy. Although for com-munity care a principal purpose of the policy change was to gain control of expenditure on residential care, it addressed also the issue of how adult services should evolve over time towards a more mixed economy of pro-viders, and a shift in the balance of care towards home-based services. The management language of community care policy with its central concepts of purchaser–provider separation, strategic planning and care manage-ment, also referred to 'quality control', and the central objective of 'secur-ing and safeguarding the necessary quality of services' for all agencies. Both central and local authorities would play a part in 'helping to main-tain, and where necessary, improve the quality of care provided' (Depart-ment of Health, 1990). Although intrinsic quality improvements to existing services were not strongly stated in policy terms (except for mental health services), the assumption was made that changes in assessment, a wider choice of services/providers, and a planned shift in the balance of care services would lead to an improved responsiveness to service users' needs, thus improving their quality of life.

Several related aspects of the policy were seen to promote quality of community care. The first of these was to improve local authorities' capac-ity to influence the quality of services through its wider function as a purchaser in the private and voluntary sectors. The process of preparation for purchasing or arranging services was seen to entail more accurate planning around identified needs, and more explicit agreement of a contractual nature about the qualities of the service, as well as the costs. The existence of a more contractual relationship between purchasers and providers in all sectors, would provide a better means of both ensuring 'built-in' quality, and a basis for more objective evaluation of quality stand-ards, through monitoring and inspection.

In managing the purchasing process, policy guidance points to the need for SSDs 'to be aware of the quality of services which users expect', and to ensure that standards are built into service specifications. Responsibility for quality also falls to providers in their delivery of quality, through their own systems of quality assurance. The guidance acknowledges that 'a criti-cal issue in commissioning care services will be the establishment of quality standards which meet the requirements of the purchaser, the service user, and to which the service provider is committed'.

A second obvious concern with quality came with the new local authority 'arms-length' inspection units, charged with the initial task of establishing an even-handed inspection of care standards in residential care, across both the public and independent sectors. In time, it was envisaged that the inspection units would build on their experience and capacity to broaden the scope of quality inspection to take in a wider range of ser-vices, and to incorporate the inspection function into a wider process of quality assurance.

It was recognized that in the same period of implementation, new and extended inspection responsibilities for children's residential services would also be required. The authorities were asked to 'give consideration' to the implications of these separate but complementary developments. In prac-tice, this has resulted, in some areas at least, in an integrated inspection unit which carries out most – if not all – of the SSDs' inspection functions. In a few cases, a further step has been taken to locate health authority registration officers within the same team (but separately accountable), so that there is a consolidated nucleus of key people and skills who can operate across the range of adult nursing homes and residential homes in fulfilling the inspection role for community care, and providing a source of expertise in the wider aspects of quality assurance.

In creating a national policy for local authority inspection units, the question of their independence proved problematic. On the one hand, there were arguments from the independent sector to create a national inspectorate that was clearly separated from the direct influence of local service providers, seen to be capable of objective judgement, and free from vested interests. On the other hand, the setting up of a new bu-reaucratic body sat uncomfortably in the context of a general policy cli-mate which sought to reduce or at least slow down bureaucratic growth and expenditure. The policy result of this debate was to locate the in-spection units initially under 'arms-length' local authority management (normally accountable directly through the director of social services to the local authority), but to anticipate possible changes later. This compro-mise was bolstered by the creation of local advisory committees, which could include independent sector representatives, and possibly service users.

Within a year of the implementation of this policy, further changes were proposed by the government, including the relocation of inspection units' accountability through the chief executive's office to the council. Debate continues about the establishment of a truly independent quality inspectorate: the local authority needs its inspection process as a vital component in the process of controlling service quality, particularly as it starts to make wider use of independently run services as a purchaser, rather than main provider of community care. It has the management framework to accommodate the machinery of inspection, and wider quality assurance work; it is publicly accountable through elected council members and, ultimately, via ministers to Parliament. But the local authority itself remains a major provider of community care (although the independent sector is now the majority supplier of residential care), and in some eyes at least, the concern remains that local authorities are not best placed to be their own judge and jury, or to recommend service improvements to a quality standard that they may be unable to afford.

Third, in the planning of community care, as expressed through the annual publication of 'Community Care Plans', the guidance to SSDs on quality matters includes four components. There should be statements about:

- the steps they [the SSD] are taking to ensure quality in providing and purchasing services;
- how they intend to monitor the quality of services they have purchased or provided;
- the setting up and role of inspection units;
- the setting up and role of complaints' procedures.

(Department of Health, 1990)

The process of planning consultation includes a statutory requirement for the incorporation of user representatives, voluntary organizations and other bodies, to take part in the public debate about quality aspects of care, as expressed in the Community Care Plan draft, prior to its final revision and publication.

Finally, the complaints procedure may be seen as a quality element in community care policy. Legislation required new procedures to be implemented in 1991 so that a local authority would be obliged to consider representations about the discharge of statutory social services functions (or failure to do so) in respect of individual cases.

Guidance on the procedures set out several objectives designed to give the service user greater power to comment on the quality of nature of services, to be represented in doing so, and to provide a means of challenging SSD decisions. It was also seen as an additional means of giving managers and councillors information with which to monitor service performance.

Quality management in action

So what does a quality service look like? In the following sketch of a newly commissioned service, a small-scale example is offered, which draws on present thinking about quality management, and sets out some of the key features that might typify the planning and start up of a community care service.

The service is commissioned in consultation with other relevant services, and with representatives of service users and carers. Objectives and resources are clarified and a service specification produced, including quality standards, and a framework of values and general principles within which the service is expected to operate. At this stage, potential providers are invited to express any interest in running a service to the published specification. The local authority SSD considers the merits of the various interested provider organizations, including their track record in providing quality services, the compatibility of their values, their stability and their capacity to provide value for money.

A provider organization is selected and detailed planning begins; again, in close consultation with other agency and user/carer representatives. The operation of the service is worked out in greater depth, against criteria of fitness for purpose, and other standards specified, within the range of available resources.

Staff are appointed, following selection in the context of agreed specifications. References are carefully followed through. Competences and qualifications have to be sufficient and appropriate to the role and tasks of the post. The staff are balanced in terms of gender, race and culture. Induction training takes place and staff members are clear about their objectives and methods. Quality standards are made clear in the training, and personal responsibilities written down. Supervision arrangements are made and further learning opportunities agreed as a regular activity.

Specific quality assurance measures are agreed. These include: a commitment to maintain the service at standards which have status at a national level, as well as local agreement, and which fully meet all statutory requirements; agreement to internal review arrangements, as well as independent/external quality evaluation and/or regular inspection. Measures of quality include the views of service users and carers, who are adequately represented in any steering, advisory or review groups and are empowered to put forward users' comments about their level of satisfaction with the services provided. A complaints procedure is accessible and capable of responding positively to representations: it operates openly and promptly, and is used to inform service change and development. Above all, the staff group creates and maintains a culture of commitment to quality.

The service's managers carry much responsibility for initiating and maintaining quality standards. From the early planning of the service, careful attention will have been paid to ways in which standards will be set, and periodically reviewed. Key areas for planning include:

* The recruitment and supervision of personnel, who will be capable of and committed to quality, and receptive to continuous new learning.
* Workforce organization that ensures personal accountability and support through regular skilled supervision, and effective leadership.
* Internal quality review procedures in which some or all individuals take responsibility for both monitoring progress towards objectives, and for initiating improvements to quality.
* Planning arrangements for external monitoring and inspection, and perhaps including accreditation by a national standard-setting body.
* Developing measures and indicators of progress and quality that will be useful in providing reports for the organization that has commissioned the service, and with whom a contract has been agreed.
* Monitoring the physical environment against specified standards, from the state of the kitchen, through the attractiveness of the front entrance to the maintenance of the roof and the disposal of rubbish.

By the end of, say, the first year, or following a major review, how would the organization concerned know whether it has succeeded in meeting its quality objectives? Some of the answers will come from the following sources:

* External inspection and or evaluation, perhaps leading to accreditation by a national body and/or to a renewed contract with, or registration by, the local authority SSD.
* Indicators of successful outcomes for service-users, including the latter's own expressions of satisfaction with the service, as well as professional views of service quality, and representation from other agencies.
* Internal audit of quality performance against previously specified standards, and records of improvements achieved.
* A low incidence of complaints, from either users and carers, or from referring agencies, and evidence that the organization and its individual members have the capacity to respond quickly and positively to learn from complaints or other problems arising.

The example offered above deals with perhaps the easiest of the quality tasks, that of starting up a new service on a small scale. Clearly, it is a different proposition to reorientate a complete range of services within a single organization which may employ up to ten thousand people and spend above a hundred million pounds a year, as do some of the larger British SSDs.

But for community care at least, the future indicated by policy is an increasingly diverse number of providers, for whom some of the steps described in the example given might be feasible. This would apply particularly when a service is being taken over by a new managing organization (such as a trust) or when steps are being taken to replace residential care with local domiciliary or day services.

Future developments

In looking ahead to the future pursuit of quality, and in the review of current concerns, several themes emerge. First is the need to improve information about service users' satisfaction with quality. The daily contact between care workers and users provides the opportunity to do this systematically, at relatively little cost. This can be supplemented by the existing consultation process for planning, by the analysis of assessment as a further source, or by survey.

More important than merely having such information is the commitment and capacity to act upon it. Although the faith of managerialism often lies with top leadership and 'product champions', there is growing experience in industry which points to better results when, instead of tying down the provider with myriad specifications and controls, greater emphasis is placed on creating the conditions in which there is mutual commitment to quality, skilful recruitment and training, active participation in change at all levels, and encouragement of innovation.

This 'tight–loose' configuration still needs strong central leadership, and the capacity to insist on key standards, but does not asphyxiate the organization with rules and procedures.

Quality agencies

Questions about the locus and organization of quality assurance work lead on from this. At the national level, a considerable number of agencies continue to act more or less independently in producing and evaluating quality standards, but it is difficult to distinguish any particular set of service standards as a national expression of bottom-line acceptability. A few are legally required but many more are merely recommended. One objective of the *Citizens' Charter* is to cut through this mass of available material and fix on and pursue rigorously – with the aid of clear performance indicators – a small number of quality standards.

Elsewhere at central level, the Social Services Inspectorate (SSI) provides government with advice about quality standards. The SSI is a professional branch of the Department of Health, accountable in England through ministers to Parliament, and headed by a chief inspector. Its primary functions are to inspect the quality of social services, advise ministers in the formulation of PSS policy, assist its implementation, and promote high service standards. It acts as the principal means of contact between the SSDs and the Department of Health, working from regional offices in principal cities across England. (Similar inspectorates operate in Northern Ireland, Wales and Scotland, and these bodies are separately accountable to their respective secretaries of state).

The work of SSIs on quality standards is broadly two-fold: it works both to 'set, use and disseminate objective criteria for assessing quality standards in the PSS', and to measure the quality of service against quality standards, through the inspection process. Both aspects are relatively new functions of central government, which only created its inspectorate in 1985 with formal recognition of the need both to specify standards in a systematic way, and to inspect against objective criteria. The inspection division of the SSI and the SSD inspection units now undertake similar tasks, although the scope and powers of the SSI are more extensive.

The Audit Commission is also an active agency which has had much to say about quality standards of management in community care and has published several influential reports aimed at improving its management processes. The commission operates independently of government and is also the body responsible for the external audit of health services and local authorities.

A recent criticism by local authorities is that the system is now top-heavy with quality controllers – in particular, the Audit Commission, the SSI and local authority inspection units – all of whom are mainly engaged in demonstrating the quality of the end result, rather than working with providers to find better ways of building in quality at the service level. It remains to be seen whether or not the more formal activities of inspection are ultimately compatible with the more pro-active and wider processes of quality assurance.

In the training field, the lead actor on social care quality standards is the Care Sector Consortium, which is the guardian body specifying the required competencies of social and health care workers in community care. Its specifications are comprehensive (almost encyclopaedic), and represent an important quality 'floor' in determining the future skills of the trained workforce, within the scheme of National Vocational Qualifications. However, the Central Council for Education and Training in Social Work remains the leading agency with responsibilities for the training standards of most of those (social workers) who will undertake care management, and who will mostly occupy the management posts of purchasing and providing organizations. Here again the future of quality development may need to consider the coherence of different national agencies, all charged with overlapping responsibilities for similar aspects of quality.

Conclusion

When considered against the sophistication of quality management in some highly developed service and manufacturing industries, the quality content of present community care policies may seem relatively crude in its reliance on inspection processes, at the quality control end of the spectrum. The action all takes place after the event, but can, nevertheless, provide a useful feedback loop to service purchasers and providers about the quality of received services, and inform the action they need to take to restore or improve standards. In public services, however, the inspection function has continued to find favour in the eyes of policy-makers, and plays an important part in quality appraisal and relevant policy development across such services as the police, education and the prison service.

For the present, service quality in community care is hard to measure, because it is a highly subjective idea and purchasers, providers and users may all have a different perspective of what really counts. Lagging behind the leading edge of quality assurance in manufacturing industries, the public sector response to these issues in community care has been initially to proliferate a mass of detailed quality standards and to install tighter inspection and monitoring arrangements at the 'quality control' end of the system. These measures have to stand as proxies for the users' view of adequate quality while the agencies develop more systematic ways of finding out what their users see as both the important elements, and levels of acceptable quality.

Ann James, in a Department of Health (1992) report, suggests that this should be seen as a healthy initial stage, but leading quickly to a lighter touch approach. A later phase might emphasize quality culture, which thrives on a smaller rule book and on the commitment and responsiveness of a skilled workforce, to get quality right. Where the demands for services heavily exceed resources, however, quality is likely to be under continuing pressure.

Perhaps one of the main values of the present quality assurance initiatives is in raising awareness of the quality issues, through the greater information about prevailing quality standards that is generated, so that the debate about quality and quantity can be better informed. Its other main potential is in focusing the energies of the workforce towards clearer objectives, and in providing a stimulus for organizational learning and innovation.

References

Department of Health (1990). *Community Care in the Next Decade and Beyond: Policy Guidance.* London: HMSO.

Department of Health (1992). *Committed to Quality.* London: HMSO.
Department of Health/Social Services Inspectorate (1991). *Purchase of Service: Practice Guidance and Practice Materials for SSDs and Other Agencies.* London: HMSO.
Maxwell, R.J. (1984). Quality assessment in health. *British Medical Journal, 288*: 1470–72.

Further reading

British Quality Association (1987). *Guidance on the Interpretation of BS5750: Part Two. With Reference to Social Care Agencies.* London: BQA.
Brook, R. (1989). *Managing the Enabling Authority.* London: Longman/LGTB.
Centre for Policy on Ageing (1984). *Home Life: Code of Practice for Residential Care.* London: Centre for Policy on Ageing.
Department of Health/Social Services Inspectorate (1989). *Homes Are for Living In.* London: HMSO.
Department of Health/Social Services Inspectorate (1990a). *Caring for Quality: Guidance on Standards for Residential Homes for People with a Physical Disability.* London: HMSO.
Department of Health/Social Services Inspectorate (1990b). *Caring for Quality: Guidance on Standards for Residential Homes for Elderly People.* London: HMSO.
Department of Health/Social Services Inspectorate (1992a). *Caring for Quality: Guidance on Standards for the Residential Care Needs of People with Learning Disabilities/ Mental Handicap.* London: HMSO.
Department of Health/Social Services Inspectorate (1992b). *Caring for Quality in Day Services.* London: HMSO.
Department of Health/Social Services Inspectorate (1992c). *Caring for Quality: Guidance on Standards for the Residential Care Needs of People with Specific Mental Health Needs.* London: HMSO.
Department of Health/Social Services Inspectorate (1993a). *Caring for Quality: Guidance on Standards for Short Term Breaks.* London: HMSO.
Department of Health/Social Services Inspectorate (1993b). *Caring for Quality: Standards for the Residential Care of Elderly People with Mental Disorders.* London: HMSO.

8 The consumer role

Jim Monach and Len Spriggs

It is one of life's more surprising ironies that the 1980s was a decade in which the New Right mounted a sustained attack on the foundations of the Welfare State, while at the same time government, reflecting New Right thinking, endorsed the value of giving those who use welfare services a much more significant say in their planning and delivery. At first sight, this seems an unholy alliance between icons of the Left such as Freire (1972), advocating the oppressed taking power to alleviate their oppression, and those of the Right like Friedman (1980), arguing the beneficence of a free market system which has in recent history been most associated with the creation of wealth at the expense of those with only their labour to sell. In the limited space available to us, we will attempt to demonstrate the difficulties which inhere in the terms in which this debate is constructed, and that what counts in the event is the means whereby principle can be converted to action, and users of services come to have a central role in community care (Williams, 1992).

Meanings

George Bernard Shaw (1987) anticipated the backlash to come when he wrote 'all professions are a conspiracy against the laity'. When the professions held their greatest sway, there was little debate about what to call those who used their services. Those who used mental health services were 'patients', whether or not they were receiving active treatment; although community-based professions bidding for autonomy from the medical profession would use the term 'client'. Just as social workers and community nurses sought to emphasize their independence through language, those on the receiving end of services have more recently acknowledged the importance of words in seeking to choose their own descriptor.

'User' is often adopted for its apparent value neutrality, although others reject it for this very reason, i.e. it avoids confronting issues of power, or are concerned at its implied link with illicit drug use. 'Survivor' appeals to those who emphasize the importance of recognizing the damage done by the conventional 'system', as in the organization Survivors Speak Out.[1] Some ex-users prefer the term 'recipient', which also conveys the sense of powerlessness in the face of services (Lawson, 1991). 'Consumer' has gained little popularity beyond official documents and the MINDLINK organization,[2] which grew out of the MIND psychiatric services 'consumer network'. It is suggested that 'consumer' pretends to be apolitical, because it ignores the reality that services often do not offer realistic choice among alternatives, as several supermarkets on the high street are said to do (Potter, 1988). The role of a retailing manager in the redesign of community care services, Sir Roy Griffiths has been ironically noted as marking this failure to acknowledge the importance of power. However, Ralph Nader's seminal work on consumer power was predicated on the analysis that monopolistic industries frequently distorted the market to their advantage and the disadvantage of the consumer. Nader might have been talking about the introduction of the purchaser–provider split within the National Health Service (NHS), and the introduction of the internal market, when he pointed out the limitations of consumerism; the public has 'never been supplied the information nor offered the quality of competition to enable it to make effective demands through the market place' (Nader, 1973). The other key failure of the analogy with commerce is that the high street retailer does not involve its customers in the planning and design of services; involvement only comes at the point of sale. This situation of passive choice at the delivery stage only has value given a wide range of choice as on the high street. The 'customers' of community care do not have this choice.

There are those who prefer to use the term 'mental patient' for ironic effect, in seeking to emphasize the extent to which those who are receiving services are subject to stereotyped categorizations by professionals (Chamberlin, 1988). The same usage can be seen in the context of Patients' Councils (Gell, 1990). There can be no doubt that there is no single term yet available which is universally acceptable and implicitly acknowledges the serious concerns of power, choice, status and value. We will adopt the term 'user' in this chapter, while accepting its limitations.

The other broad area in which the meaning of terms is of particular importance is in relation to the processes and ways of working which arise from different perceptions of how services should be organized to best reflect the interests of those who use them. Self-help has the longest history: 'the root of all genuine growth in the individual' (Smiles, 1890). Adams (1990) describes this as 'a process . . . comprising people coming together or sharing an experience or problem with a view to individual

[1] Survivors Speak Out, c/o Peter Campbell, 33 Lichfield Road, London NW2 7NX.
[2] MINDLINK, c/o 22 Harley Street, London W1N 2ED.

and/or mutual benefit'. It has been used less recently for the suspect connotations of being independent of other forms of help, and potentially, a cheaper alternative for the welfare agencies. Empowerment has come to be accepted as the appropriate alternative, seen by Croft and Beresford (1990) alongside 'involvement' as the key welfare word of the 1990s. Empowerment involves people becoming able; as Adams (1990) says, 'to take control of their circumstances and achieve their own goals, thereby being able to work towards maximising the quality of their lives'. The distinction which is the key to this usage is that between 'enabling', denoting skills imparted by another, and 'empowering', denoting the taking of control by the user of services; the role of the professional in this context is to contribute to a setting in which this can happen most effectively.

'Advocacy' is becoming a significant focus and approach to user involvement in services, although there are a number of ways in which the term is used. The simplest conceptualization is as a process by which service users, individually or in groups, make their views and interests known to service providers. 'Advocacy and self-advocacy promote the growth of the individual and enable the process of valorisation' (Lawson, 1991), that is, the acquisition or reinforcement of a socially valued role or status. Advocacy is inextricably linked with principles of normalization and social role valorization (Wolfensberger, 1983) and its concern to reverse the process of devaluation of people with disabilities by changing the way services are delivered and self-definitions constructed: 'we learn to define ourselves by the roles and diagnoses given to us by psychiatrists, take them into ourselves and feel helpless to influence our own lives' (Lindow, 1990). The advocacy movement challenges the power of professionals, not only in terms of service delivery but in the conceptualization of disability itself. Important distinctions in this context are 'self' and 'citizen' advocacy, which will be considered separately.

Involving users: A trend in social policy

The move towards involving users in the planning and delivery of services reflects an established trend towards greater user participation. Since the late 1960s, an increasing number of reports and statutes have enshrined this expectation: the Seebohm Report (1968) and subsequent reorganization of social services in 1970; the introduction of the community health councils in 1974; the first Griffiths' Report on the health service in 1983; the Disabled Persons Act 1986; the Children Act 1989; the National Health Service and Community Care Act 1990. These are but a few of the significant statements of policy which have advocated and required the active involvement of users in the planning and delivery of services. A parallel development has been to encourage the development of services at a neighbourhood level, whether in community nursing (Cumberlege, 1986), social services (Seebohm, 1968) or health services (Griffiths, 1988). The rationale for locating services locally is the facilitation of communication between service planners and providers and service users.

It is one thing to advocate such a change of emphasis, and quite another to implement it: 'Much of the fashionable rhetoric about integration is hot air. Disabled people remain a marginalised and stigmatised group . . . nevertheless rhetoric has a certain power. It has begun to change social attitudes' (Beardshaw, 1988). In fact, describing the development of the Nottingham Patients' Councils Support Group, Colin Gell (1990) observes:

> . . . overall, the major success [of NPCSG] has been in changing the attitudes of mental health workers who are now more ready to consult users before services are developed. Increasingly, users are being involved in projects as a matter of course, rather than as something innovative, or as an afterthought.

Beardshaw identifies the attitudes which are seen as obstructive by disabled people who have 'come to see health professionals' traditional "caring" approach as oppressive and patronising. They experience problems of communication and rigid approaches to treatment that fail to adapt interventions to individual needs.' The 'new' emphasis on user participation and involvement can be seen as a reaction to the paternalistic style of service delivery and the real lack of service often experienced by some of the most disadvantaged and devalued people in British society.

This change of emphasis towards consumer choice and citizen involvement may be seen, increasingly, across all the public services (Citizens and Patients Charters, 1991, 1992). The twin roots of this change were economic and political. In the wake of monetarist theories, with the renewed emphasis on the beneficial effects of competition, came a shift to greater diversity in the supply of services, and a shift away from state to voluntary and private provision. The belief is that consumers will be best served by ensuring that they have choice; their choices will drive standards upwards. This belief seems to survive the evidence of the effect of choice and private provision on the health care available to the poor in the United States of America. As legislators they have become more convinced of the value of funding a national system of health care from taxation, the United Kingdom has been eroding that principle. Political pressures have come from quite disparate sources: the principles of the free market and a diminishing role for the state in welfare as in all areas of social life: a burgeoning movement of user and advocacy groups, demanding the right to have a real say in the planning and delivery of services. User involvement is clearly an idea whose time has come, although there is much concern that the transition to practice may not be so straightforward.

User involvement in practice

As Beresford (1992) points out, user involvement is no longer simply a 'good thing': users' organizations demand it, legislation requires it and much has been written about it (Harding and Upton, 1991). One of the central policy aims of *Caring for People* (Department of Health, 1989) is to give people more say in the services they use. At the heart of the National Health Services and Community Care Act 1990 is the individual consumer: 'Promoting choice and independence underlies all the Government's proposals' (ibid.). Care management and assessment are seen as 'the cornerstones of quality care' and 'the rationale for this reorganisation in the delivery of care is the empowerment of users and carers' (DoH/SSI, 1991). Local authorities providing social services are required to consult with service users, users' and carers' organizations, and the black and minority ethnic communities in a number of spheres: the creation of community care plans; assessment and care management proposals; arrangements for the commissioning and purchasing of services and contract specifications; advisory mechanisms for the work of independent inspection units; complaints procedures ensuring proper attention to problems of quality or access.

There are particular difficulties in relation to the involvement of black and ethnic minority communities and users in service planning and delivery (Baxter *et al.*, 1990; Christie and Blunden, 1991). Many have pointed out the need to avoid a 'colour blind' approach in order to ensure that services are genuinely accessible and appropriate to all in a multicultural society, as is required by *Caring for People.*

Although there is considerable scope for user and carer involvement in developing community care, there remain two major difficulties. First, it remains firmly in the hands of the local statutory authorities to do the 'involving'. Users' and carers' organizations have no independent rights to representation and involvement, and assessment only happens at the instigation of the local authority. Second, users' and carers' organizations have many, and increasing, demands made upon them, and usually limited resources to meet those demands. These lead to widespread scepticism about the reality, meaningfulness and extent of user involvement. A recent survey found only 29 per cent of statutory authorities with written policies in relation to user involvement (Croft and Beresford, 1990). Massie (1992), for example, points out that the Disabled Persons (Services, Consultation and Representation) Act 1986 laid the foundation for consultation: people with disabilities were to have their views sought, to be consulted about services, to receive a written statement of services to be provided and, most importantly, to be given reasons why appropriate services would not be provided and the right of appeal. In 1991, the government decided that these dormant provisions would not be implemented as they were superseded by the general provisions for the right of consultation given in the National Health Services and Community Care Act 1990. The key difference is that under the provisions of the 1986 legislation, the individual with the disability would lead the process of assessment; however, the 1990 Act leaves lead responsibility to the authority, makes no provision for the representation of those who are unable to put their own case, nor does it require the local authority to be accountable by giving reasons for not providing a service. People with disabilities, it is argued, will therefore remain at the margins, not at the centre.

Similar reservations have been registered in relation to people with learning disabilities. Research by Simons (1992) in this field has demonstrated the gap between the rhetoric of participation and reality in four crucial areas of statutory rights to involvement. Service users had many criticisms of the services they used, but few had ever used a formal complaints procedure for two basic reasons: the probable adverse consequences of any complaint and the possible damage to their relationships with carers – 'the sub-culture of service settings discourages moaning and being miserable' (Simons, 1992), which is what making a complaint was felt to represent. There is now a lengthy experience of Individual Programme Planning (IPP) for people with learning disabilities in assessment and care planning. This has not been an unqualified success, with users reporting not being listened to, their 'key worker' doing all the talking, feeling tested and no action following. Simons reported that the IPP environment did not encourage users to assert their point of view, and that there appeared to be an unconscious rationing process at work whereby what was needed was defined in terms of what was available. Involvement in the work of inspection units is likely to be minimal if they concentrate on registration and policing minimal standards rather than quality evaluation, where users are likely to have the greatest expertise and feel most comfortable. Finally, users had mixed experiences of consultation over community care plans, and noted instances in which their views differed from the approach adopted without any explanation being offered. An example of this was abandoning contract work viewed by workers as demeaning and anachronistic but valued as constructive activity by users: the implicit message was that users' views did not count. *Changing the Balance: Power and People Who Use Services* (Thompson, 1991) illustrates the difficulties which users themselves experienced in this process.

The issue of resources is crucial to this process of consultation. One reason for not involving users in planning services is that they may discover what they are entitled to, and would therefore ask for it (Simmons, 1992). Recent government ministerial statements appear to endorse the view that this is a reason for limiting consultation (*Guardian*, 1 July 1993). The concern and cynicism that the context of declining resources creates is highlighted by Jean Collins (1992) of Values into Action. 'It is paying lip service to the Act. If no more money is in the pot then users are no better off' (Stone, 1992). The evidence of the first round of community care plans is that local authorities can produce documents acceptable to the Department of Health containing long lists of desired developments with no indication of their relative priority to each other, nor to existing services, let alone the 'priorities' they suggest for savings in the many authorities working to reduced budgets. 'There is a general feeling among voluntary groups and users' groups that consultations conducted in an uncertain financial climate are a waste of time' (Stone, 1992). Objectively, it could be argued that consultation is even more essential then, but the real experience is that authorities do not consult about reductions of service; these crucial decisions never get into the process at all.

The process of consultation is often criticized for the way in which documents are often written in 'officialese' and never reach the majority of users in a form in which they could be understood, and upon which they could meaningfully comment: 'In our area the problem was that they had not consulted about how to consult' (Stone, 1992). A survey of elderly people (Peace *et al.*, 1992) showed that care is still predominantly service-led, rather than needs-led, and that the role of service providers, as seen by many users *and* professionals, was that of managing scarce resources – hardly conducive to notions of choice or empowerment as envisaged by *Caring for People*. Similarly, the Wakefield Case Management Project found 'a serious discrepancy in the needs of clients and the resources available' (Richardson and Higgins, 1990).

Advocacy: Empowering users

The concept of advocacy as we understand it today was first developed in the USA and Europe in relation to 'mental handicap' and in Holland in relation to 'mental health'. Advocacy is used in a variety of ways, and in practice it can be difficult to separate issues of advocacy from processes of user involvement and participation. However, a key aspect is the extent to which the advocacy movement challenges the power of professionals, not only in terms of service delivery but in the conceptualization of disability itself. In the field of mental health, self-advocacy is often ideologically linked with the 'anti-psychiatry' movement, but as Campbell (1990) points out, although there are links the two cannot be seen as synonymous. Without considering paid or legal advocacy and the various national voluntary organizations representing users' interests (see Brandon, 1991a), there are various layers to the advocacy movement ranging from citizen advocacy's exclusive focus on the individual, through the reformist approach of the self-advocacy movement and their participation in service planning and delivery to the more radical critique offered by the 'separatist' wing of the user movement (see Chamberlin, 1986).

Citizen advocacy is a form of lay advocacy developed in the USA, designed to promote the rights, interests and acceptance of people with learning disabilities. This approach has been extended to other groups, including people suffering from dementia (Sang, 1986). Citizen advocacy emerged because many people who use long-term services are unable, for whatever reason, to speak for themselves, or have been denied the opportunity to develop the skills and confidence to do this. The growth of citizen (and self-) advocacy is in essence a response to the powerlessness and devaluation experienced by users of health and social services, the denial of their basic human rights, and their exclusion from the communities in which they live. Citizen advocacy is founded on the belief that all people have value and rights, no matter what their disability, and its objective is to empower those who have been kept powerless and/or excluded.

The central element of citizen advocacy is the notion of a partnership between an individual who has a disability (the partner) and another who does not (the citizen advocate), who is independent, unpaid and, in Wolfensberger's terms, 'valued' (i.e. non-disabled). Citizen advocates develop a one-to-one relationship with their partners and represent their partners' interests as if they were their own. An essential ingredient of the partnership is that the advocate recognizes the qualities of the 'devalued' partner. The substantial and growing number of citizen advocate offices in North America and in the UK work to the principles set out by Wolfensberger (1983) and O'Brien (1987).

Butler and Forrest (1990) identify four key characteristics of successful citizen advocacy. First, the individual advocate must be independent of any service provision used by the person with disabilities in order to avoid any conflict of interest, and likewise the advocacy office must be independent of service-providing agencies. Second, and central to citizen advocacy, is the one-to-one relationship between the advocate and partner. Citizen advocacy is explicitly aimed at upholding the basic human rights of the devalued individual: it is not collective advocacy. Third, a citizen advocacy relationship should strive to be a long-term and continuous one. However, short-term 'crisis' advocates may be recruited in special circumstances, such as the transfer of a number of hospital residents into the community. Fourth, the advocate's commitment and primary loyalty must be to their partner, not the advocacy office nor the partner's family if there is a clash of interests.

The advocate will thus play a variety of roles. Butler and Forrest (1990) discuss two main strands in the advocacy relationship: the instrumental and the expressive. The *instrumental* role is essentially a problem-solving one, where the advocate might, for instance, help facilitate access to health and social services, help their partner obtain welfare benefit, represent their partner in negotiating a care plan and speak on his or her behalf.

The róles are many, just as the relationship is open-ended; they might even include enabling significant life choices to be made such as getting married. The *expressive* role involves meeting the emotional needs of their partner, and offering friendship, sharing family and friends, as well as providing support in a crisis. 'The crux of CA [citizen advocacy] lies in the nature . . . of the relationship between the devalued person and the advocate' (Butler and Forrest, 1990). Its function is to include the 'excluded', and by so doing empower people with disabilities and enable them to obtain, so far as possible, the rights of citizenship which ordinary society takes for granted. Detailed descriptions of citizen advocacy in practice are 'A Powerful Partnership' (Butler *et al.*, 1988) and 'Including the Excluded' (Forrest, 1986).

Self-advocacy, in contrast, is about people becoming their own advocates, and speaking for themselves, perhaps initially with the support of others (Gell, 1990). A 'partner' may become a self-advocate because of the confidence gained from the citizen advocate relationship. Indeed, there is some commonality in function and origin between citizen advocacy and self-advocacy. Self-advocacy is concerned with 'both people's personal and political needs, offering warmth, friendship and support as well as teaching social skills and representing people's interests in local and national affairs' (Croft and Beresford, 1990); they, too, can be involved in a range of activities. It is perhaps important, therefore, given the role envisaged in statute, to distinguish, as Croft and Beresford do, between consumerism and self-advocacy:

> Consumerist approaches to involvement tend to be service provider led, those for self advocacy, user led. These different philosophies reflect real tensions between service providers and users over involvement. Each is concerned with meeting their own needs. These are not the same.

Self-advocacy and citizen advocacy are about empowerment; consumerism is about consultation and information gathering. Unlike citizen advocacy, self-advocacy is not rooted in a clearly formulated set of principles developed by concerned professionals, but rather, as Campbell (1990) says, in the 'Personal experiences of [the psychiatric] system which too often fails to meet human needs . . . and . . . feeds into society's prejudices by segregating service recipients, and promoting negative stereotypes'. Lindow (1990) makes the point that self-advocacy is about 'seizing the right to define ourselves'.

There has been a significant increase in the number of self-advocacy groups in the field of learning disabilities, and there are now more than 200 such groups affiliated to People First; more than half adult training centres now have one. The difficulty People First faced in 1992 becoming registered as a charity in the UK is indicative of the problems which the welfare establishment has in coming to terms with the reality of empowering service users. Patients' Councils have had an equally significant role in promoting user involvement in the mental health field (documented by Gell, 1990), the role of which is to support users in speaking for themselves rather than speaking for them. Self-advocacy has the important function of facilitating collective action as well as making it easier to be assertive without 'upsetting staff' and to develop confidence and learn new skills.

> Self Advocacy requires a commitment from the user involved. To have such a commitment users need to value themselves . . . to become aware of their rights and responsibilities . . . to develop skills of problem solving and decision making and develop assertiveness skills.
> (Walsh, 1985)

Sutcliffe (1990) also emphasizes the importance of education and skill development in this process.

Because of the value attached to independence, it is sometimes suggested that the greatest threat to advocacy schemes comes from the benign paternalism of professional workers. A parallel might be drawn with the field of anti-oppressive practice in social work, where an analysis of the development of a truly anti-racist perspective of practice arguably only came with the strength of black social work organizations (Central Council for Education and Training in Social Work, 1991). Sang (1988) points out that these skills should be learned independently of the professional agencies which disempowered users in the first place. Marsh and Fisher (1992) place their faith in training to avoid professionals paying lip service to principles of advocacy while in reality exploiting the users' lack of a voice to claim that 'we do this already'. Brandon (1991a) is less sanguine, arguing that it is virtually impossible for paid professionals to act as advocate because they are usually paid by the organization against whom users may seek redress. In the Wakefield Case Management Project, professionals saw themselves acting as advocates as well as case managers: a dual role which undermines the notion of independent advocacy (Richardson and Higgins, 1990).

It is important, however, not to dismiss the contribution of professionals too lightly. It is usually acknowledged that developments in self-advocacy benefit from the support of professionals, at least initially. Workers have the skills to promote the development of new organizations, can access resources and provide 'insider' information. Campbell (1990) shows this ambivalence clearly: professionals played a significant role in helping Survivors Speak Out become established and gain the necessary skills, but, however unintentionally, the self-confidence of professionals can lead them to play a dominating role. For these reasons, Judi Chamberlin fundamentally doubts that professionals can ever engage in a genuine partnership with people with disabilities:

> Both psychiatric survivors and radical mental health workers propose an ideology of empowerment and autonomy: it remains to be seen if these two groups can overcome their historic differences, including class and power, to promote these ideals for all.
>
> (Chamberlin, 1988)

The commitment of professionals to advocacy, in any form, is to be welcomed, as long as they fully understand what it means, but it is important to recognize the dangers of such commitment and be wary of advocacy groups being too closely embraced by service providers. The development of People First was inhibited by too close ties to statutory services. As Sang (1988) argues, independence is the key if advocacy is to promote real change. If government policy is aimed at empowering users, as it claims, then independently funded advocacy is essential. Campbell (1990) asks the sobering questions: 'How much is really up for change? How far are those with power prepared to share it with recipients? And how compatible is the Government's concept of consumerism with the developing philosophy of Self Advocacy?'

Making it work

Putting the principles of user involvement into action requires both information and education. Access to quality information is crucial, if choice is to be exercised as a means to empowerment. The authors' current research into the views of users of mental health services confirms the small proportion of users who feel they were given enough information about their treatment (Monach and Spriggs, in prep.). Beresforth *et al.* (1990) are quite explicit: 'information is power'. They argue that the information needs of users should have priority over those – in descending order of priority – of care workers/case managers, service managers, and policy makers. Shared information is essential for effective care plans, which should be jointly written, in plain English, and agreed as part of an open dialogue. Information should be seen as a resource which enables users to improve the quality of services rather than, as is largely the case now, a part of the process of mystification, and therefore disempowerment of service users.

Controlling information is crucial to the control of knowledge and, therefore, power. As Brandon (1991a) notes, professional practice mixes care and control and the exercise of both can devalue and depersonalize users. This may be seen in the context of confidentiality, which is

> ... presented to them as being necessary for their care and the co-ordination of services, is preserved as part of the caring relationship

and broken for the same reason. This double-bind situation 'sub-merges' users, they become unable to challenge the breach of confidence if they wish to gain access to certain services.

(Smith, 1989)

Without denying the relevance of expert knowledge, this should be seen as one layer among many (Ramon, 1991). There is the danger that professional 'interpretations' might involve a distortion of users' perceptions of their own needs (McKnight, 1981). The structured inequality of the provider–user relationship does not exist in a vacuum but reflects and reinforces the oppressive character of a wider, class-based society in which many identifiably different groups suffer institutionalized disadvantage. Such groups not infrequently internalize such negative stereotypes, as Meade and Carter (1990) argue in the case of ageism and the elderly. Professional and user profiles usually differ significantly, particularly along axes of class, age, income, race, gender and disability (Miller and Rose, 1986).

The very term 'community' may be unhelpful in focusing attention on the disadvantages to be addressed, by conflating the individual and the social. Indeed, Dalley (1983), from a feminist perspective, suggests that 'communality' may be a more appropriate term, as it embraces recognition of the disproportionate burden borne by women consequent upon care in the community, and the inappropriate individualization of service delivery. Perhaps, ironically, one of the radical approaches suggested to care management is service brokerage. This argues for individual control of resources and greater choice about the services consumed (Mason, 1992). However, service brokerage, it could be argued, reflects and reinforces the welfare ideology of the self-interested individual, competing for scarce resources in the marketplace. 'All for each, each for all that is society [and community]: each for himself, and thus each against all, that is individualism' (Lukes, 1973). In addition, early evaluations of service brokerage even cast doubt on its practical effectiveness (Beardshaw and Towell, 1990). Socially structured inequalities need to be addressed at a structural level, although their effects may be modified at an individual level. Smith (1989) sees the resourcing of user groups as a means of challenging prevailing ideologies as well as sharing information and changing working relationships.

Both users and professionals in such an endeavour will need training to engage fully in changed patterns of working. This training will not be easy, as such changes require 'a substantial attitude and skill shift' (Brandon, 1991b). Attitudes are notoriously difficult to shift, whatever the circumstances: 'A major skill lies in developing structures which encourage open systems so that staff and users feel listened to and valued: able to make positive contributions' (ibid.). It is equally important that action takes place at a community level to broaden and strengthen efforts directed to self-help, partnership and participation, as illustrated by Meade and Carter (1990), if there is to be an impact on public health policies, services and structures.

Creating partnership

There are many obstacles to user involvement in the delivery of care: services encourage dependency and marginalization; the controlling character of the medical model of disability encourages distance from users; professional colonization of 'progressive' approaches to practice. For example, Brandon (1991b) points to the significant danger that normalization will become yet another form of 'professional evangelism'. Psichiatria Democratica in Italy represents one of the most radical attempts to build a non-stigmatizing service for those with mental health problems, with true community participation (Ramon, 1988); however, its critics still see it as flawed, as it is predicated on medical leadership – the Italians, too, are having to look outwards for ideas on involving users more fully. It is perhaps inevitable that professionals will resist this threat to their hegemony and point to the dangers of devalued people receiving deprofessionalized (i.e. poor-quality) services (Wilkinson and Freeman, 1986), or criticize the user groups as non-representative and unreliable or simply creating more work for already overstretched services. As Brandon (1991a) asserts, user involvement will only become a significant force if 'users take more power and influence as well as being given it'. Marsh and Fisher (1992) helpfully illustrate the principles upon which partnership practice can evolve, but in doing so demonstrate the number of competing interests which have to be negotiated. Current government policy reflects a narrow view of user involvement in assuming that this can be achieved simply through the mechanisms of consumer choice and contracts. This is an integral part of the purchaser–provider split and the concept of care management. However, early indications are that contracts within this context are not increasing user choice of service (Common and Flynn, 1992).

As long as community care is inadequately funded, superficially conceptualized and professional attitudes are resistant to change, creating the reality of partnership from the rhetoric of professionals and public policy is likely to be a struggle; but a challenging one in which all must engage.

References

Adams, R. (1990). *Self-help, Social Work and Empowerment.* London: Macmillan.
Baxter, C. *et al.* (1990). *Double Discrimination.* London: King's Fund.
Beardshaw, V. (1988). Aiming to be less of a client, more of an ally. *Health Service Journal,* September, pp. 994–6.

Beardshaw, V. and Towell, D. (1990). *Assessment and Case Management: Implications for the Implementation of 'Caring for People'.* London: King's Fund.

Beresford, P. (1992). No longer simply a good thing. *Community Care,* 26 March, Supplement, p. ii.

Beresforth, M. *et al.* (1990). *Whose Service is it Anyway? Users' Views on Coordinating Community Care.* London: Research and Development for Psychiatry.

Brandon, D. (1991a). *Innovation Without Change.* London: Macmillan.

Brandon, D. (1991b). The implications of normalisation work for professional skills. In Ramon, S. (ed.), *Beyond Community Care.* London: Macmillan/MIND.

Butler, K. and Forrest, M. (1990). Citizen advocacy for people with disabilities. In Winn, L. (ed.), *Power to the People: The Key to Responsive Services in Health and Social Care.* London: King's Fund.

Butler, K. *et al.* (1988). *Citizen Advocacy: A Powerful Partnership.* London: National Citizen Advocacy.

Campbell, P. (1990). Mental health self advocacy. In Winn, L. (ed.), *Power to the People: The Key to Responsive Services in Health and Social Care.* London: King's Fund.

Central Council for Education and Training in Social Work (1991). *Setting the Context for Change.* London: CCETSW.

Chamberlin, J. (1986). The case for separatism. In Barker, I. and Peck, E. (eds), *Power in Strange Places.* London: Good Practices in Mental Health.

Chamberlin, J. (1988). *On Our Own.* London: MIND.

Christie, Y. and Blunden, R. (1991). *Is Race on Your Agenda?* London: King's Fund.

Collins, J. (1992). *When Eagles Fly.* London: Values into Action.

Common, R. and Flynn, N. (1992). *Contracting for Care.* York: Community Care/ Joseph Rowntree Foundation.

Conservative Central Office (1991). *Citizens' Charter.* Cm. 1599. London: HMSO.

Conservative Central Office (1992). *Patients' Charter.* London: HMSO.

Croft, S. and Beresford, P. (1990). *From Paternalism to Participation: Involving People in Social Services.* London: Open Services Project.

Cumberlege, J. (1986). *Neighbourhood Nursing: A Focus for Care. Report of the Community Nursing Review Team.* London: HMSO.

Dalley, G. (1983). Ideologies of care: A feminist contribution to the debate. *Critical Social Policy,* 8: 72–81.

Department of Health (1989). *Caring for People: Community Care in the Next Decade and Beyond.* Cm. 849. London: HMSO.

Department of Health/Social Services Inspectorate (1991). *Care Management and Assessment: Summary of Practice Guidance.* London: HMSO.

Forrest, A. (1986). *Citizen Advocacy: Including the Excluded.* Sheffield: Sheffield Citizen Advocacy, Aizlewood's Mill, Sheffield S3 8GG.

Freire, P. (1972). *Pedagogy of the Oppressed.* Harmondsworth: Penguin.

Friedman, M. (1980). *Free to Choose: A Personal Statement.* Harmondsworth: Penguin.

Gell, C. (1990). User group involvement. In Winn, L. (ed.), *Power to the People: The Key to Responsive Services in Health and Social Care.* London: King's Fund.

Griffiths, R. (1983). *N.H.S. Management Inquiry: Report to the Secretary of State for Social Services.* London: HMSO.

Griffiths, R. (1988). *Community Care: Agenda for Action.* London: HMSO.

Harding, T. and Upton, A. (1991). *User Involvement in Social Services: An Annotated Bibliography.* London: National Institute of Social Work.

Lawson, M. (1991). A recipient's view. In Ramon, S. (ed.), *Beyond Community Care.* London: Macmillan/MIND.

Lindow, V. (1990). Participation and power. *Open Mind,* April/May, pp. 10–11.

Lukes, S. (1973). *Individualism.* Oxford: Blackwell.

McKnight, J. (1981). Professionalized service and disabling help. In Brechin, A. *et al.* (eds), *Handicap in a Social World.* London: Hodder and Stoughton.

Marsh, P. and Fisher, M. (1992). *Good Intentions: Developing User Orientated Services Under the Children and Community Care Acts.* York: Community Care/Joseph Rowntree Foundation.

Mason, P. (1992). The litmus test. *Social Work Today,* 11 June, pp. 12–13.

Massie, B. (1992). Empty wrappings. *Community Care,* 26 March, Supplement, p. i.

Meade, K. and Carter, C. (1990). Empowering older users. In Winn, L. (ed.), *Power to the People: The Key to Responsive Services in Health and Social Care.* London: King's Fund.

Miller, P. and Rose, N. (eds) (1986). *The Power of Psychiatry.* Cambridge: Polity Press.

Monach, J. and Spriggs, L. (in prep.). *Self-perceived Requirements for Community Care Amongst Users of Mental Health Services.* Sheffield: Sheffield Hallam University.

Nader, R. (ed.) (1973). *The Consumer and Corporate Accountability.* New York: Harcourt Brace Jovanovich.

O'Brien, J. (1987). *Learning from Citizen Advocacy Programs.* Atlanta, GA: Georgia Advocacy Office.

Peace, S. *et al.* (1992). *Elderly People: Choice, Participation and Satisfaction.* London: Policy Studies Institute.

Potter, J. (1988). Consumerism and the public sector. *Public Administration,* 66: 149–64.

Ramon, S. (1988). *Psychiatry in Transition.* London: Pluto Press.

Ramon, S. (ed.) (1991). *Beyond Community Care: Normalisation and Integration Work.* London: Macmillan/MIND.

Richardson, A. and Higgins, R. (1990). *Case Management in Practice: Reflections on the Wakefield Case Management Project.* Leeds: Nuffield Institute, University of Leeds.

Sang, B. (1986). Advocacy and people with dementia. In *Living Well into Old Age,* Appendix 1, pp. 26–30. London: King's Fund.

Sang, B. (1988). The independent voice of advocacy. In Brackx, A. and Grimshaw, C. (eds), *Mental Health Care in Crisis.* London: Pluto Press.

Seebohm, F. (1968). *Report of the Committee on Local Authority and Allied Personal Social Services.* Cmnd 3703. London: HMSO.

Shaw, G.B. (1987). *Doctor's Dilemma.* Harmondsworth: Penguin.

Simmons, D. (1992). Needs *v* cash. *Community Care,* 26 March, Supplement, pp. vi–vii.

Simons, K. (1992). Who counts? *Community Care,* 26 March, Supplement, pp. iv–v.

Smiles, S. (1890). *Self Help with Illustrations of Conduct and Perseverance.* London: John Murray.

Smith, H. (1989). Collaboration for change. In Towell, D. *et al.* (eds), *Managing Psychiatric Services in Transition.* London: King's Fund.

Stone, K. (1992). Unfounded fears. *Community Care,* 2 April, p. 7.

Sutcliffe, J. (1990). *Adults with Learning Difficulties: Education for Choice and Empowerment.* Milton Keynes/London: Open University Press/ National Institute for Adult and Continuing Education.

Thompson, C. (ed.) (1991). *Changing the Balance: Power and People Who Use Services.* London: National Council of Voluntary Organizations/ Community Care Project.

Walsh, P. (1985). Speaking up for the patient. *Nursing Times,* 1 May, pp. 24–6.

Wilkinson, G. and Freeman, H. (eds) (1986). *The Provision of Mental Health Services in Britain.* London: Gaskell.

Williams, J. (1992). User involvement: Working together? Paper presented to the *Conference on Schizophrenia: Innovations in Clinical Practice,* Sheffield Hallam University, July.

Wolfensberger, W. (1983). Social role valorisation: A proposed new term for the principle of normalisation. *Mental Retardation, 21*(6): 234–9.

Section 3

Models of care

9 Residential services

Andy Alaszewski and Wai-Ling Wun

Introduction

In this chapter, we consider the development of residential care in the community as an alternative to institutional care. First, we discuss the development of models of care by first focusing on the development of services for children and then on adult services. Then, we examine the ways in which the models of residential services have been converted in practice by focusing on two research studies. The first study is based on the development of ordinary living for children with profound learning disabilities in ordinary housing. The second examines the type of services provided for adults discharged from hospital in the West Midlands to illustrate the range of different support which has developed.

Models of residential care

Residential care for children

Prior to the Second World War, there were two parallel streams in the development of residential services for children. Residential care for children with a learning disability was mainly provided by the state within large institutions or mental handicap hospitals, in which children were cared for alongside adults. Other children tended to be cared for by voluntary agencies such as Dr Barnardo's, whose initial commitment to providing services for children came from taking responsibility for destitute children in the growing Victorian industrial conurbations. These agencies provided residential care in institutions often known as 'village developments' which had 'cottage' homes for children.

The institutional model first began to break up in the general child care services. A key influence was the psychoanalytical studies by such researchers as Burlingham and Freud (for a discussion of this development, see

Heywood, 1978). Burlingham and Freud studied the large state nurseries which looked after many children during the Second World War. They argued that this type of care had a very damaging effect on young children, as it disrupted the bond between the child and his or her mother. These studies had an important influence on the Curtis Committee, which was appointed in 1945 to investigate the provision of care for children who were deprived of a normal home life. The Committee accepted that growing up in institutions damaged children and that: 'The lack of the mother's fondling cannot of course be entirely made good, but something must be provided which gives the child the feeling that there is a secure and affectionate personal relationship in his life' (cited in Shearer, 1980: 12). These studies had two, rather contradictory effects. They resulted in a shift in emphasis from institutional to community-based residential facilities and, simultaneously, a marginalization of the role of residential care. Care in families was best and residential care could, at best, provide a poor imitation of real family life.

After the Second World War, the newly established Children's Departments began to develop alternatives to large institutions. One model which was particularly popular in the North West of England was the group home. Although some authorities adopted the group home model, in others the emphasis was on family placement, either through foster families or adoption. Initially, the preference among authorities and their professional staff tended to be pragmatic – family placement tended to be cheaper. However, within the mainstream child care services, families were increasingly seen as not only the *best* place to provide care but also the *only* place to provide care (see discussion by Morris, 1984). Within social services and social work, residential care was marginalized – it was a necessary evil. Residential placement was seen as a short-term expediency, either to assess a child or prepare a child for family placement. Only children who were difficult to place tended to be left behind and became semi-permanent residents.

Initially, the development of services for children with a learning disability lagged behind the development of mainstream services. While Children's Departments were moving away from institutional care in the 1950s and 1960s, health authorities were actually expanding the institutional provision for children with a learning disability. Indeed, while the 1971 White Paper *Better Services for the Mentally Handicapped* (DHSS, 1971) recommended a substantial reduction of institutional provision for adults, it recommended only a small reduction of hospital provision for children (see Table 1).

In the 1960s, researchers such as Tizard and his colleagues challenged the accepted view that children with a learning disability required the specialist medical and nursing facilities of institutions, and demonstrated that these children could and did benefit from care within mainstream

Table 1 Planning figures for services for people with a learning disability in England and Wales compared with existing provision in 1969

Type of service	Places for children (age 0–15 years)		Places for adults (age 16+ years)	
	Required	Provided	Required	Provided
Residential care in the community (including short-stay):				
• in local authority, voluntary or privately owned residential homes	4900	1800	29 400	4300
• foster homes, lodgings, etc.	1000	100	7400	550
Hospital treatment:				
• for in-patients	6400	7400[a]	27 000	52 000[a]
• for day patients	2900	200[b]	4900	500[b]

Source: DHSS (1971: 42).
[a] NHS beds allocated to those with a mental handicap; [b] estimated.

child care facilities such as group homes (see, e.g. Tizard, 1964; King et al., 1971). However, as services for children with a learning disability began to catch up with mainstream child care services, so these mainstream services had moved on and away from residential care. However, the newly developing services for children with a learning disability could not dispense with residential services. There were still a substantial number of children in mental handicap hospitals, and many children coming into the care of local authorities had such severe handicaps that family placement was not considered feasible at the time. These new services needed a rationale for and a model of residential provision.

Normalization provided a basis for a distinctive model of care. Normalization is a philosophy of care for people with disabilities, which developed in Scandinavia at the end of the 1950s and was based on a critique of institutional care. Advocates of normalization argued that life in institutions was grossly abnormal. Institutions increased and added to the disabilities of their inmates. People with a disability had a right to a service which gave them access to normal life experiences, thus enhancing their skills and abilities (see, e.g. Race, 1987).

This model of residential care found its best expression in the Jay Committee, which reported on mental handicap nursing and therefore needed to consider the alternative to nursing in the mental handicap hospitals. The Jay Committee based its model on an ideological commitment to the rights of people with a mental handicap. In particular, the committee stated that 'mentally handicapped people have a right to enjoy normal patterns of life within the community' (Jay, 1979: para. 89a). The committee was critical of all purpose-built residential facilities, even small hostels, as it felt that such purpose-built facilities tended to be institutional in nature. To ensure people with a learning disability could experience everyday life, the committee argued that all residential facilities should be provided in 'ordinary houses, suitably adapted for those with additional physical handicaps' (ibid.: para. 135). The committee felt that 'such houses [should] be in specially adapted private houses' (ibid.: para. 114).

In its discussion of the organization of the residential facilities, the committee stressed the importance of the normal experiences of everyday life. The committee felt that 'mentally handicapped people should be able to develop a daily routine like other people' (ibid.: para. 91h). The committee saw the provision of normal life experiences as a central feature of the new residential units.

> The small unit which we envisage is a place where residents and staff live together as a unit, a place where meals are cooked, washing-up is done and tradesmen are seen. In such small homes . . . the child will experience as normal a life as possible . . . the contribution of those in the surrounding neighbourhood will be of high importance, and neighbours, shop-keepers and friends will play their part. We want the children to see the milkman and, however small they are, to be taken out shopping. This means that the social unit is one in which the staff are not enclosed but share many aspects of daily living with the children.
>
> (Jay, 1979: paras 116 and 119)

The Jay Committee's prescription formed the basis of work by subsequent committees. For example, the Barclay Committee's report on the role of social workers emphasized the importance of the social worker–resident relationship in residential care and argued that each resident should have a key worker who would plan and coordinate their services. The committee, implicitly drawing on psychoanalytic theories of child development, identified a second key relationship for each child – a parenting relationship:

> For satisfactory emotional growth and development every child needs, we think, the unconditional commitment of at least one person (usually mother or father, or both). For a child in residential care this person may be someone outside a residential establishment or foster home. Sometimes he or she will be found only within the residential setting. Each child in long-term care needs such a person and one of the tasks of the key workers is to make sure, when ever possible, that a committed adult is available to the child.
>
> (National Institute for Social Work, 1982: 70)

The Wagner Committee on residential social work clearly felt that the role of key worker and surrogate parent should be combined:

The continuity which comes from having consistent attention from staff whom an individual can come to know well and trust, is an important aspect that has to be planned, managed and coordinated. This is one reason why the development of residential 'key workers' as a means of establishing some continuity of care should be encouraged.
(National Institute for Social Work, 1988: 63)

Thus in the 1980s, there was a broad agreement among policy makers that children with a learning disability should have the right to the same experiences as other children and in particular a close relationship with a significant adult. When these experiences could not be provided within a family, then the next best was in ordinary houses in which the pattern of relationships and activities was modelled on those of an ordinary household.

Developing services for adults

There are important similarities and differences between the development of residential services for children and adults with a learning disability. Until the late 1960s, the bulk of residential care for both groups was provided in mental handicap hospitals and for both groups there has been a shift to residential care within the community. However, there has been a difference in the speed of the change and models of care adopted. For children, the move from institutional care to ordinary housing and family placement is now complete. For adults, the transition from institutional to community-based facilities has been slower and there is still considerable debate about the most appropriate models of care and funding relationships.

The difference in the pace of change for the two groups related to the numbers involved, the different characteristics of the two groups and to the level of central government concern. There were far more adults in institutional care in 1969: 52 000 adults compared with 7400 children. The numbers of children in hospital fell rapidly in the 1970s, to 3900 in 1977 and approximately 2000 in 1981 (DHSS, 1980). Much of this reduction was created by sleight-of-hand – as the children grew older, they were simply reclassified as adults. The reduction in the adult hospital population, however, was slower. The 1971 population of 52 000 adults was reduced to 45 400 by the end of 1979 and to 22 100 by 1991. A substantial part of this reduction was achieved by discharging people from hospital and developing alternative provision within the community. Between 1979 and 1991, an additional 20 400 residential places were created in community-based facilities (Department of Health, 1992).

In the institutions, children and adults with a learning disability tended to be treated in the same way – the emphasis was on their common needs, which were a product of their common disability. With the development of community-based services, there has been an increased emphasis on generic services. There has been a tendency to emphasize the similarities between people with a learning disability and other citizens. This has been particularly marked for children. The common needs of children (i.e. protection and close bonds with parents) have meant that models of care developed in mainstream child care have been easily adapted for children with a learning disability. For adults with a learning disability, particularly if their disability is severe, associated with a physical disability and/or challenging behaviour, it is not so clear and obvious how and in what ways ordinary services could and should be adapted, and in particular what balance should be struck between independent living and protection or supervision by staff. The type and level of risk need to be explicitly considered (Alaszewski and Manthorpe, 1991).

The commitment of central government to change has also been different. The Jay Committee's (1979) view that it was unacceptable for any child to grow up in an institution such as a mental handicap hospital was accepted by ministers and was supported by researchers such as Shearer (1980). The secretary of state made a public commitment to move all children out of hospital by the beginning of 1985 (DHSS, 1981). There has been no equivalent 'moral' pressure on ministers to move adults with a learning disability. This has reinforced the impediments created by the large numbers and debates about the alternatives.

Initially, the main model for community-based services for adults was the purpose-built authority-funded hostel. This model was described in the White Paper *Better Services for the Mentally Handicapped*, although it was called a home rather than a hostel:

> ... residential homes for the mentally handicapped are a permanent substitute family home for most of the residents, even though they keep in touch with their own families and visit them as often as possible. The staff and residents become a substitute family group. The home should be homely. Homes of this kind will supply much of the residential care needed. They should be small, and usually have residents of both sexes. For adults, 25 is now normally the maximum for a single home, and 20 the maximum for children; many may be smaller. Most adults should have single rooms, and no rooms have more than four beds. Plenty of space for recreation is needed, indoors and outside. Residents should use local parks and sports grounds, and shops. In such surroundings a family atmosphere can be created, where individuals can develop within a small group and with their own interests and possessions.
>
> (DHSS, 1971: paras 161 and 163)

Progress in the 1970s in developing community-based services was relatively slow. Local authorities were reluctant to make the investment and take on the long-term commitment of 25-bed, purpose-built hostels. In 1976, to assist local authorities, the Department of Health developed a system of joint funding through which National Health Service (NHS) funds could be transferred to local authorities. The scheme was modified by the DHSS in 1983 to include not only joint funding for specific projects but also a 'dowry' scheme in which money was tied to patients; that is, when a health authority transferred responsibility for the care of a specific individual who was in a long-stay hospital, it could also transfer the money which had been used to fund that person's care in hospital. The emphasis on moving patients out of hospital and the associated financial incentives resulted in a two-tier service – a 'Rolls Royce' service for people discharged from hospital with cash dowries and a cheaper service for other clients. There was little incentive and few resources for local authorities to provide residential support for adults living in families that were experiencing severe stress.

In the 1980s, central government attempted to increase the speed of deinstitutionalization. It fostered research into different models of care and introduced new forms of funding. To guide the development of community services in 1980 and beyond, central government fostered and evaluated a number of demonstration or pilot projects (for a summary of research findings, see Robbins, 1993). In England, the DHSS provide £17 million between 1984 and 1985 for a demonstration programme to initiate twenty-eight pilot resettlement projects spread over a wide range of geographical areas and client groups (Knapp *et al.*, 1992). In 1983, the Welsh Office developed a parallel initiative for people with a learning disability. The All-Wales Strategy provided a set of principles to guide service planning and a source of money for new services development (Beyer *et al.*, 1992). The All-Wales Strategy endorsed the concept of ordinary living in ordinary houses as the preferred mode of residential care:

> Support staff should be available to help run a range of accommodation . . . [which] . . . should be in ordinary houses and made available from local housing stock. This means that new purpose-built hostels, or hospitals or units should not form part of the new patterns.
>
> (Welsh Office, 1983)

The pressure to provide community-based services in the 1980s led to the development of alternative methods of funding. In addition to the direct funding of the health services and social services and the transfer of NHS resources to social services via joint funding and 'dowries', the government also increased funding to the voluntary and commercial sectors. The voluntary sector benefited from housing grants which the Housing

Corporation made available to housing associations to provide special needs accommodation; the commercial sector benefited from the increase in social security funding of claimants living in residential and nursing homes. The varying sources of funding stimulated a patchwork of providers and types of provision. In her review of residential provision for people with learning disabilities undertaken for the Wagner Committee, Atkinson (1988) identified six separate types of residential accommodation: residential accommodation for children, hostels, group homes, ordinary housing, residential accommodation for 'people with special needs', and private and voluntary homes. These can be further subdivided. For example, group homes can be subdivided in terms of size and pattern of staffing, while private accommodation can vary from residential home, through lodging to independent living in rented accommodation.

Having created this patchwork of services and funding, the government is now attempting to re-establish control by creating a lead agency and giving prime responsibility for funding to one agency, Social Services. By the end of 1992, local authorities were required to have in place agreed strategies with health authorities for placements of people in nursing homes, and hospital discharge assessments and plans in their community care plans. However, these plans tend to be position statements couched in broad terms and do not document resource commitments or outline responsibilities (Wistow *et al.*, 1993).

The reforms are designed to control the escalating costs of community care by giving the main responsibility for the purchasing of residential care in the community to one lead authority. However, they are deliberately designed to enhance choice and efficiency by creating competition between various providers of residential services. Given the inevitable patchwork of services and models, there is a danger that purchasers will tend to buy the cheapest rather than the best. Without information on quality and consumer preferences, purchasers will tend to equate value for money with cheapness. It is important to evaluate alternatives so that quality can be balanced against cost.

From theory to practice

Ordinary living for children: The case of Barnardo's Croxteth Park Project

In this section, we discuss the development of one particular service, Barnardo's Croxteth Park Project for children with a profound learning difficulty. The main features of the Croxteth Park Project have already been well documented (Alaszewski and Ong, 1990), and we will concentrate on those distinctive features of the project which make it a model for other residential services.

The Croxteth Park Project was based on and develops a distinctive model of care. This model of care was in part derived from the traditions of mainstream child care services, with its emphasis on residential care as a short-term means to an end:

> Residential Care is not an end in itself . . . the majority of children in Barnardo's residential care are placed for more sustained periods with the objective of enhancing their capacity either to return to their own families long-term or to prepare for living with a substitute family or to achieve a greater degree of independence and fulfil-ment in less dependent forms of 'sheltered' or residential care.
>
> (Barnardo's, 1981)

Within the project, this child care tradition was explicitly linked to the normalization philosophy. The project was seen not only as a way of pro-viding residential care, but also as a means for enhancing the social image of the residents and providing them with the opportunities to experience everyday life.

> We were particularly influenced by his [Wolfensberger's] view that service providers should value people with a mental handicap so that they could compensate for the effect of previous stigmatisation and devaluation. It was particularly important that people with a mental handicap should have their social roles enhanced through, for ex-ample, the use of positive imagery.
>
> (Alaszewski and Ong, 1990: 11)

This concern with enhancing the image of the children permeated the project. It influenced the choice of families. Many residential facilities are established in low-cost properties, such as large Victorian houses. This type of accommodation is cheap to purchase, but it is also often located in run-down neighbourhoods. Barnardo's deliberately chose to locate their project in an expensive, newly constructed housing estate. The Divisional Director described the choice of housing in the following way:

> We are going to care for the most problematic of children in this field, in an ordinary setting and, through moving them into an even better setting, we enhance them. Doing it in a nice place, in a posh estate reflects well of the kids.

The integration of the child care tradition can best be seen in the most distinctive feature of the project – the caring relationship which Barnardo's fostered between the children and the care staff. Each child had a link worker who was his or her child's prime carer. The link worker was expected to develop a close bond with their child and to foster a surrogate parent relationship. Barnardo's described the importance of this caring role in the following way:

> The aim will be to ensure as far as possible that each child always has one adult offering him exclusive attention . . . The child/adult contact

will not be haphazard, but will be consciously planned as part of a curriculum developed individually for each child.

The development of the link worker role was a conscious rejection of some of the traditions of professional practice, in particular the tradition that care staff should maintain a degree of detachment from their clients. The divisional managers wanted to use the emotional attachment that developed between link worker and child as part of the therapeutic process. The link worker was not only to be the child's key worker but was also expected to act as substitute parent. The divisional managers wanted link workers to develop an emotional bond or attachment with the child in their care. The manager drew on the work of Bowlby (1979) and Fahlberg (1979). Using a psychoanalytical perspective, Bowlby argued that it is essential for the mental health of a young child, that that child experience a warm, intimate and continuous relationship with his or her mother. The development of the strong bond between each child and his or her link worker was a central feature of, and played a key role in, achieving the therapeutic objectives of the project. The Project Leader described the function of the attachment in the following way:

> The children coming to our service had, as a result of living in long-stay institutions, experienced few opportunities to build up close relations with significant adults . . . They had come to equate physical and verbal contact with care tasks such as feeding and dressing, and had little experience of close and loving interaction for its own sake . . . We viewed emotional investment of staff in a child as beneficial for a child's personal growth and ability to develop social interaction. We asked workers to 'contractually' engage themselves in a committed relationship with the child and take on the responsibilities of a surrogate parent.

The attachment was a means of preparing the child for family placement. The divisional managers felt that once a child had developed an attachment to an adult, that child would be able to learn to transfer this attachment to another adult, such as a foster parent. The link worker had to accept that although they would, for a time, be the most important person in that child's life, other adults could and should take over that responsibility. The Project Leader described this aspect of the link worker's role in the following way:

> The growth and development of the child as the result of this relationship [with his or her link worker] was not an end in itself, but was considered to be a step towards building a future with meaningful relationships. This means concretely that the link workers were working towards rehabilitating the children with their natural families, finding foster families for them or other suitable community

provision. As a logical consequence of the application of the normalisation philosophy . . . family life was considered a desirable goal and staff had to learn to cope with transferring the emotional relationship to families.

We have documented elsewhere (e.g. Alaszewski, 1992) how an innovative programme can be fully evaluated. This can be done in a number of ways. For example, we monitored the progress of the children admitted to the project over a period of six years. An independent psychological report summarized the children's progress in the following way:

> . . . when the children were reassessed after six months in the Project they showed substantially improved performances. In this six-month period most of the children showed improvements of between 20 per cent and 33 per cent in the various areas of assessment. After this initial increase in performance, the children continued to make progress but their improvements were more limited. Given the profound handicap of the children and poor medical prognosis this was remarkable and almost certainly related to the excellent quality of care given within the Project.
>
> (Lovett, 1990: 224–5)

Residential services for adults: The West Midlands Resettlement Study

In this section, we discuss the findings of a survey undertaken by the Centre for Research and Information into Mental Disability at the University of Birmingham on behalf of the West Midlands Regional Health Authority into the residential care provided for adults in the West Midlands Region who have been resettled from hospital (Wun and Cumella, 1993). This survey provides an excellent insight into the range of different facilities available and the different experiences of residential care.

The research was based on a survey of 177 people discharged from mental handicap hospitals between 1 April 1985 and 1 April 1991. Their age ranged from 18 to 87 years and the average was 46 years. The people resettled had high levels of need. Over half of them were socially impaired, compared with 40 per cent in the Darenth Park study (Korman and Glennerster, 1990), and 39 per cent had challenging behaviour.

These former patients were resettled in accommodation which varied from independent living to hostel accommodation in which more than twenty people lived in the same unit. The majority (83 per cent) were resettled in facilities with a high staff: client ratio, in which staff provided 24-hour support and supervision. Most (76 per cent) lived in facilities which used the concepts of 'ordinary life' as the basis of their care philosophy and were based in ordinary housing which had been adapted. However, the size of these facilities varied. The units managed by local authorities and the private sector tended to be larger (mean size 15 and 14 clients, respectively) than the units managed by health authorities and voluntary agencies (mean size six clients). There was also a difference between the facilities in rural and urban areas. In some of the suburban areas, the facilities had been developed by the health authorities in the mid-1980s, and provided units for four clients or less and were located near shops, etc. The facilities in the urban areas tended to comprise units which had often been established in the 1970s. The units developed in ordinary housing were developed in the mid-1980s, but most were close to other special needs residential facilities.

Felce's framework for evaluating the nature of different residential facilities can be used as a framework for presenting the results of the survey. Felce and Perry (1993) suggest that quality of residential facilities can be judged in terms of the extent which users of the facilities:

- have opportunities to experience ordinary community life and be part of the community they live in
- are able to maintain a social network and enjoy a variety of social relationships
- are able to participate in the full range of activities of ordinary life and to grow in experience and competence over time
- have opportunities for choice and are able to exercise choice.

All the units catered for the residents' basic needs and in all of them residents had a reasonable physical environment which enabled them to have their own private space and facilities for storing their own possessions. Though some homes had beautifully decorated communal areas, residents' rooms were sometimes rather bare. Some residents appeared to maintain the institutional practice of hiding their personal possessions and not even displaying them in their own rooms.

Having experienced the 'ordinary life' ethos of the units, all the residents participated in running their home by undertaking some domestic chores. The level of involvement varied with the size of home, with the residents in the larger units participating less. In some cases, this reflected a positive choice by residents, as they had chosen a larger unit because they had to do fewer chores. The level of participation was highest in those facilities managed by voluntary agencies and lowest in those facilities managed by the private sector. The staff also shared in the residents' lives; for example, in most homes (64 per cent), the staff took their meals with the residents. In some of the private homes, the staff wore uniforms. The rationale for this was 'hygiene and economy'. Home managers were proud of this practice.

All the facilities offered opportunities for community participation. In the month prior to the research visit, most residents had used local facilities such as shops, hairdressers, pubs and cafés, half had used leisure facilities such as clubs, cinemas and theatres, and a third had attended church services. Some residents occasionally went to restaurants for meals and used sports facilities. Most had a holiday at least once a year. Those residents who lived in smaller facilities, especially those managed by health authorities, made the most use of community facilities, whereas the residents in larger local authority hostels made least use of these facilities.

Again all the facilities gave their residents a degree of autonomy, though the level of autonomy depended on the type of activity involved. The residents could usually exercise a degree of choice over the way they spent their time and the activities they performed, but staff tended to exert more control over activities which involved money or the security of the home. In most homes there was an unresolved tension between enabling the residents to make choices and take risks and ensuring their safety and protection.

It has been argued that moving into the community does not necessarily increase community participation, as living in specialist residential units and other settings offers little opportunity for the development of relationships outside the unit (Dossa, 1992). This was the case in the West Midlands study. Although those people living in homes in the suburbs seemed to have more social contacts outside the home than those living in inner-city or rural areas, the overall participation rates were low; indeed, for some, these had deteriorated following discharge from hospital. A study of 108 hospital residents undertaken by the hospital resettlement team on behalf of the project, indicated that 96 per cent had known family but only 66 per cent had contact with their family, and 80 per cent had one or more friends but only 40 per cent had regular contact with these friends. In contrast, resettled individuals had narrower social networks but tended to use them more effectively. Of the 178 resettled individuals, 92 per cent had known family and 72 per cent had contact with their family, and 64 per cent had one or more friends and 46 per cent had regular contact with these friends (see Tables 2 and 3). Discharge from hospital meant that residents' potential networks of relatives and friends were smaller but were used more often.

Table 2 Contacts with family members (percentages)

	Visits by family		Contact other than visits	
Frequency	Hospital	Community	Hospital	Community
Weekly	23	22	5	17
Monthly	13	15	5	15
Less often	30	35	50	34
Never	30	20	35	26
No known family	4	8	5	8

Table 3 Contacts with friends (percentages)

	Visit friends		Visits by friends	
Frequency	Hospital	Community	Hospital	Community
Weekly	5	11	6	11
Monthly	10	11	9	8
Less often	30	19	28	27
Never	35	23	37	19
No known friend	20	36	20	35

Forty-six residents were willing and able to speak to the research team about their experiences and views. All these residents preferred living in the community facilities, although a third wanted to move on to less restricted and controlled environments. They generally appreciated the improvements in their physical environment, although some of the residents with physical disabilities felt that living in ordinary housing created problems, as they found it difficult to manoeuvre their wheelchairs. Most residents felt that the relationships in their home worked well and they got on well with other residents and the staff, although some residents did feel that if they did not 'fit' in they would be sent back to hospital and that any friction between residents would be magnified because of the small size of the homes. There were some examples of friction; for example, one resident felt that staff intruded when the staff's relatives or friends visited her home. Occasionally, there were problems with neighbours who were not welcoming.

The residents seemed to enjoy being involved in the running of their homes. Most seemed to enjoy and were proud of the ways in which they contributed. A small minority complained they had too much to do, although under-involvement seemed more of a problem. Over a third complained that they were often bored. Although the residents found they had more control over their own lives, this control was still limited. One elderly resident said she received £1 each week to attend a club and 50 pence to buy crisps and that staff bought all her clothes and personal possessions. She never went shopping, 'because I don't have the money'.

The only area in which the residents expressed anxiety or concern was social relations. A number of residents said they felt lonely and had lost contact with friends since their move from hospital. Many of these friendships had lasted for many years. One person who was physically handicapped and used a wheelchair said that when he was in hospital he could wheel himself round the grounds to see his friends, but in his new unit 'nobody comes round'. He said that the unit staff had tried to invite neighbours round but none of them had responded. Another resident had returned several times to his former hospital to visit friends, but they had now moved and the hospital staff were unable or unwilling to tell him where they had gone and he was very upset about this.

The move to living in the community not only provided residents with more opportunities and choice, it also increased their knowledge of everyday living and increased their expectations. Of seventeen individuals who wanted to move on, four wanted to return to their family; the majority wanted to move to a less restricted environment with more personal space, such as their own house or flat.

Conclusions

In the last twenty years, there has been a major shift in government policy regarding residential care. Hospitals are no longer seen as acceptable for either children or adults with a learning disability, and the government is committed to developing residential facilities within the community.

Following a period of experimentation in the 1970s and 1980s with alternative models of residential care, facilities such as Barnardo's Croxteth Park Project have demonstrated that even the most profoundly disabled people can be cared for and benefit from living in small units located in ordinary housing in the community. As a result of this and related demonstration projects, living in ordinary housing is now the generally preferred model.

Given the investment in other facilities located in the community, such as local authority hostels, and given the variety of funding, there is now a variety of different types of facility with different management structures. The current development of a managed market for residential facilities will make social services departments the main purchasers of residential care. However, the impact of this change will depend on the relationship between social service departments and the real consumers of health care. It is clear that these consumers prefer living in ordinary houses within the community in the least restricted environment possible. However, these type of facilities remain in short supply. If the new system is resource-driven rather than needs-led, then social services departments may be tempted to purchase facilities at the lowest cost, perhaps even in traditional institutions.

References

Alaszewski, A. (1992). The Croxteth Park Project. In Robbins, D. (ed.), *Community Care: Findings from the Department of Health Funded Research, 1988–1992.* London: HMSO.

Alaszewski, A. and Manthorpe, J. (1991). Measuring and managing risk in social welfare: A literature review. *British Journal of Social Work, 21*: 277–90.

Alaszewski, A. and Ong, B.N. (eds) (1990). *Normalisation in Practice*. London: Tavistock/Routledge.

Atkinson, D. (1988). Residential care for children and adults with mental handicap. In Sinclair, I. (ed.), *Residential Care: The Research Reviewed*. London: National Institute for Social Work.

Barnardo's (1981). *Intensive Support Unit for Mentally Handicapped Children*. Liverpool: Barnardo's North West Division.

Beyer, S., Todd, S. and Felce, D. (1992). The implementation of the All-Wales Strategy. *Mental Handicap Research*, 4: 115–40.

Bowlby, J. (1979). *The Making and Breaking of Affectionate Bonds*. London: Tavistock.

Department of Health (1992). Personal social services: Provision for people with learning disabilities, England, 1979–1990. *Statistical Bulletin*, 3(6): 92.

Department of Health and Social Security (1971). *Better Services for the Mentally Handicapped*. Cmnd 4683. London: HMSO.

Department of Health and Social Security (1980). *Mental Handicap: Progress, Problems and Priorities*. London: DHSS.

Department of Health and Social Security (1981). *Mental Handicap: Priorities for the 1980s*. Press Release, 81/272.

Dossa, P.A. (1992). Ethnography as narrative discourse: Community integration of people with developmental disabilities. *International Journal of Rehabilitation Research*, 15: 1–14.

Fahlberg, V. (1979). *Attachment and Separation: Putting the Pieces Together*. Michigan, IL: Michigan Department of Social Services.

Felce, D. and Perry, J. (1993). Refining measures of the quality of community residence for people with learning disabilities. In Robbins, D. (ed.), *Community Care: Findings from the Department of Health Funded Research, 1988–1992*. London: HMSO.

Heywood, J.S. (1978). *Children in Care: The Development of the Service for the Deprived Child*. London: Routledge and Kegan Paul.

Jay, P. (1979). *Report of the Committee of Inquiry into Mental Handicap Nursing and Care*, Vol. I. Cmnd 1468. London: HMSO.

King, R.D., Raynes, N.V. and Tizard, J. (1971). *Patterns of Residential Care: Sociological Studies in Institutions for Handicapped Children*. London: Routledge and Kegan Paul.

Knapp, M. *et al.* (1992). *Care in the Community: Challenge and Demonstration*. Canterbury: Personal Social Services Research Unit, University of Kent.

Korman, N. and Glennerster, H. (1990). Hospital Closure: A Political and Economic Study. Milton Keynes: Open University Press.

Lovett, S. (1990). The psychological development of the children. In Alaszewski, A. and Ong, B.N. (eds), *Normalisation in Practice*. London: Tavistock/Routledge.

Morris, C. (1984). *The Permanency Principle in Child Care Social Work*. Norwich: University of East Anglia.

National Institute for Social Work (1982). *Social Workers: Their Roles and Tasks*. London: Bedford Square Press.

National Institute for Social Work (1988). *Residential Care: A Positive Choice*. London: HMSO.

Race, D. (1987). Normalisation: Theory and practice. In Malin, N. (ed.), *Reassessing Community Care*. London: Croom Helm.

Robbins, D. (ed.) (1993). *Community Care: Findings from the Department of Health Funded Research, 1988–1992.* London: HMSO.

Shearer, A. (1980). *Handicapped Children in Residential Care: A Study of Policy Failure.* London: Bedford Square Press.

Tizard, J. (1964). *Community Services for the Mentally Retarded.* Oxford: Oxford University Press.

Welsh Office (1983). *All-Wales Strategy for the Development of Services for Mentally Handicapped People.* Cardiff: Welsh Office.

Wistow, G., Hardy, B. and Leedham, I. (1993). Planning blight. *Health Service Journal,* 18: 22–4.

Wun, W.L. and Cumella, S. (1993). *Resettlement from Mental Handicap Hospital: A Report Completed for the West Midlands Regional Health Authority.* Birmingham: Centre for Research and Information into Mental Disability, University of Birmingham.

10 Day services

Steve McNally and John Rose

This chapter aims to examine recent developments in day services for a range of people whose needs may be assessed and met according to the National Health Service and Community Care Act (1990). The implementation of the Act from April 1993 is likely to have effects for everyone who works – informally or formally – to support a potentially vulnerable person in the community. It addresses the challenges which exist for professionals who are involved in providing day services to various groups of service users. We also intend to consider some of the agents for change that currently exist and are influencing developments. We will then discuss how the changes that the National Health Service and Community Care Act (1990) will bring are contributing to changes in services and examine the implications for the future.

Development of day services

Much of the current day service provision for adults with learning disabilities is based on a model of segregated day service developed in the 1960s and 1970s. These developments were generally well intentioned, attempting to provide the individuals who attended with a useful occupation and to provide respite to carers, usually parents or relatives (Roberts, 1990). These services had a variety of names, such as adult training centres (ATCs), sheltered workshops and occupational centres. The centres were often located on trading estates, isolated from many community facilities. However, this was in keeping with their role whereby users would be occupied with contract work for local industry. A variety of tasks would be and are still performed in some centres, including packing Christmas cards, despruing plastic components, and assembly tasks.

A small wage or 'pocket money' was generally paid, but this was at most no more than a few pounds each week. With contracts to be met and relatively poor staff: client ratios (one member of staff to ten 'trainees'), it is perhaps unsurprising that many centres concentrated most of their efforts into meeting their contracts. Little effort or emphasis was placed on enabling attenders to develop appropriate life skills or move on to paid work (McConkey and Murphy, 1989).

A national survey of ATCs carried out over five years and including data from 78 per cent of the centres in England and Wales found that managers saw work training as their main aim (Whelan and Speake, 1977). Approximately one-third of the ATCs saw their role as preparing people for open employment. However, less than 5 per cent of clients were placed successfully in sheltered or open employment (Owens and Birchenall, 1979). Where clients had secured a real job, only 33–50 per cent were posts related to previous training at the ATC (Whelan and Speake, 1977).

An influential report was compiled by the National Development Team for the Mentally Handicapped in 1977 which recommended a change in emphasis for the centres, from an occupational to an educational role. They recommended that the adult training centres change their name to social education centres and that the people who attend them should be known as students rather than trainees. They also recommended that at least some activities should be held in the community rather than the centre. Although many centres did start to make changes, only a few models of good practice emerged and there was little clear guidance as to what constituted a good service.

The concentration of services for large groups of people with diverse needs, on isolated sites and with poor staff:client ratios, seems to have slowed developments in many areas until recently (Wertheimer, 1987). As hospitals have closed and the emphasis has moved towards community-based provision, the importance of day services for both the personal development of service users and to provide respite for carers has increased. Adult training centres or social education centres (also known as resource and activity centres) have been described as the 'backbone' of day services to people with learning disabilities (Audit Commission, 1987).

An inspection of day services by the Social Services Inspectorate (1989) found that there had been a large increase in day centre places in the UK, from 23 000 in 1969 to 50 300 in 1986, with the most recent estimate of places being about 56 000 (Local Authority Circular No. 15, 1992). This represents a considerable amount of investment in resources. Even though the Social Services Inspectorate found a number of models of good practice, they also reiterated a number of criticisms of traditional day services. These included the segregated nature of services and also the low level of 'through put' to more integrated services, possibly associated with the generally poor levels of individual planning for clients in many centres. These recommendations confirmed earlier reports of centres becoming 'silted up', with their clients being 'stuck' (Shearer, 1986; Wertheimer, 1987).

These criticisms have been echoed to some extent by the centre users themselves. Jahoda *et al.* (1989) questioned users of Scottish day centres who were glad to have somewhere to go during the day, but they felt that – in the long term – traditional day services did not make a positive contribution to their lives and they said that they would prefer ordinary jobs.

Current models of day service

Recently, there has been considerable interest in day services, with a number of publications advocating a range of service developments. It is therefore hardly surprising that many centres have developed to serve a number of different, sometimes incompatible, purposes (Seed, 1988, Harper, 1989; Rose and Adamson, 1990; Woolrych, 1990) and that standards of current day provision are variable (Mittler, 1990; Beyer *et al.*, 1994).

For example, Seed (1988) found seven distinct models of day centre functioning (e.g. work, social care and further education models). However, even though centres may have attempted to work specifically towards one model, the competing needs of users and service systems almost invariably resulted in centres attempting to fulfil a number of different functions. Here we will review briefly some of the areas that have been the subject of the greatest interest over recent years, and examine some additional pressures on current services.

Adult training centres

Adult training centres have offered a range of activities and experiences to clients, whom they have served with some success. Too often the ATC has been the only service available to the school leaver. Community care policies stress that services have a strong value base, are non-institutional and offer choice to users. Day centres are likely to be part of service provision for some time to come.

However, we anticipate the development of more varied community-based provisions from day centres. Smaller groups of clients should spend a higher proportion of their time in integrated settings; this would benefit clients and be consistent with accepted models of service accomplishment (e.g. O'Brien, 1985). The caveat here is resources, but successful providers will demonstrate positive outcomes for clients and attract funding.

Purchasers and providers of day services have a crucial role to play in preparing people for employment by equipping them with the necessary skills for work. These skills will be general and interpersonal in nature (Department of Health, 1992).

Resource centres

Some of the most innovative developments have involved attempting to provide services in the community. A number of articles (e.g. Bender,

1986; Harper, 1989; Allen, 1990; Nelson, 1990; Cassam, 1991) have described services which involve outreach work in community facilities or in the homes of users. These authors describe, or have attempted to provide, services which are independent of buildings, except as an office base that could be shared with other organizations (Wertheimer, 1987). Staff members are used to facilitate access by service users to all types of community facilities such as colleges, places of work, leisure centres and shops. Staff will also work with people in their own homes, if that is where the activity would normally take place.

This style of organization has many attractions, encompassing features such as community presence which are essential for a good service. However, the little research that exists in this area suggests that staffing implications are greater for an outreach service (Allen, 1990). This will no doubt slow developments towards this type of model.

Continuing education

Education has been high on the agenda for many day services since the National Development Team Report of 1977. In many areas where this was seen as essentially a centre-based activity, there have been a number of interesting developments recently. Not only is education seen as an integral part of the curriculum in many day centres, but opportunities are being created for individuals and groups to develop their skills in colleges of further education, both generally (Sutcliffe, 1990) and with specific goals in mind, such as developing work skills (King's Fund, 1984).

The transition from school to work is a sensitive phase for individuals attaining adulthood and for their families. Consideration should be given to this and to the individual need for continuing education. This may take the form of attendance at a further education college or be delivered by education or social services staff at the day centre or in an appropriate community setting.

Learning the skills of independent living will be very important; opportunities to practise skills such as shopping, cooking and dealing with money (e.g. budgeting for housekeeping, using bank accounts and paying bills) will be valuable. Students must have access to education for personal and social development. Social skills can be modelled and taught directly in a structured way or be learnt as an integral part of other educational, vocational or leisure activities. People may need support in acquiring the skills to form relationships, including close friendships, in which they can express their emotions.

A number of specific vocational training courses exist. For example, Jones (1992) describes a further education course which provides a 'step by step' approach towards full-time open employment. This course is known as the computer workshop and concentrates on using and teaching skills associated with new technology. MENCAP's Pathway Employment Service is one of the major initiatives in South Wales. It utilizes a number of schemes (e.g. Job Introduction, Sheltered Placement) to integrate people into open work settings. At the Sheffield 'Intowork' scheme, an employment development officer liaises with employers to find paid work opportunities for clients living in health authority accommodation. Four job trainers are supporting twenty people, helping them to develop the skills to work independently (Sutcliffe, 1990).

Employment and work

Work is culturally important in achieving full participation and equality in society. Historically, a segregated system of training and employment has developed for people with disabilities, whether physical or intellectual. The unemployment rate for 'economically active' people with a disability was estimated at 27 per cent for men and 20 per cent for women, compared with 11 and 9 per cent of men and women, respectively, in the whole population (Floyd, 1990). People with a learning disability have always been over-represented in the unemployed population.

The benefits of participation in meaningful, paid employment in integrated settings has been recognized for some time. A person with a physical or intellectual disability has the same right as others to valued, rewarding and unsegregated work – 'real work' with pay and security, as well as the opportunity to work with non-disabled peers (King's Fund, 1984). There is a growing acknowledgement that even people who experience a severe learning disability can benefit from job opportunities (Woolf, 1990).

Recent research has shown that day opportunities for occupation are developing in a number of different ways (Seed, 1988; Woolrych, 1990; McConkey and McGinley, 1992). Some authorities have approached the issue of work directly. For example, Blake's Wharf was funded by Hammersmith and Fulham Social Services, who – rather than develop another day centre – provided funds for a comprehensive employment service (Porterfield and Gathercole, 1985). This aimed to find employment directly for people without them necessarily attending a day centre. Other schemes such as the sheltered placement scheme developed by the Shaw Trust have enabled people to be employed in a wide range of jobs (Porterfield and Gathercole, 1985). This enables individuals to be employed and paid a full salary, some of which is paid by the employer, but with a contribution from the state, depending on an assessment of the productivity of that individual compared to other workers.

Other specific initiatives have been developed, such as workers' co-operatives and sheltered work groups (King's Fund, 1984; Wertheimer, 1985; Sikking, 1986, Gathercole, 1987). These schemes enable people to become involved in 'real work', often of high status, and provide some opportunities for interaction with people without disabilities and also allow them take a share of the profits of their endeavours. The EXCEL employment agency at Hornsey, London specializes in finding work for people with disabilities, as well as older people and women who are returning to the jobs market. Employees are paid the proper market rate for the job, while funding is provided by large, mainly private sector organizations, who pay a fee to the agency for each employee. Another model is that of work placement officers being employed in day centres, with the expectation that most, if not all, of the people with a mild learning disability will leave day centres for either work or work experience placements (Woolf, 1990; Shanly and Rose, 1993). Some individuals have found employment with the help of a job coach, whereby a person is provided with the assistance of a coach to help them develop the necessary skills for doing the job and if necessary for staying in it.

These initiatives, combined with highly systematic teaching strategies (e.g. Beyer and Kilsby (undated); Brown *et al.*, 1987; McLoughlin *et al.*, 1987; Rusch, 1990), have started to open up the possibility of work with people who have more severe or profound disabilities and special needs. The Real Jobs Project – which is a coalition of the National Development Team, Training in Systematic Instruction and the Joseph Rowntree Trust – is a recent supported employment innovation (Wertheimer, 1992). It is designed to stimulate job opportunities for people with (severe) learning disabilities and to increase public awareness of their needs.

Unfortunately the numbers of more disabled individuals being enabled to take advantage of work opportunities remains small (Kregal and Wehman, 1989; Shafer *et al.*, 1990; Wertheimer, 1992).

Leisure and recreation

The area of leisure is, in the sense of what we choose to do rather than what we must do, an important indicator of our quality of life. Traditionally, people with a learning disability have tended to spend a high proportion of their time on passive, solitary leisure pursuits, such as watching television or doing puzzles (McConkey *et al.*, 1981; Browne and Singh, 1990; McEvoy *et al.*, 1990). For many, this impoverishment of social life has often been most prominent during the evenings and weekends (Martin and Parrott, 1989). While many people live in the community, they may be home-centred in leisure terms, not having the opportunity to participate in community activities. Browne and Singh (1990), while seeking to assess the need for a community leisure initiative in Tower Hamlets, discovered that 84 per cent of respondents (service users) wished to take part in leisure activities not pursued at the time of the study. There is evidence from the USA (Benz *et al.*, 1986) which points to problems of access to community-based day and leisure programmes for clients living in residential nursing homes. Outside opportunities are more likely to be offered to clients who are young, male and mobile.

Various 'leisure links' schemes have been described. A volunteer is introduced to a services user and helps the person to use mainstream clubs and other facilities. Partnership projects involving professionals and volunteers (who have received appropriate training) can be effective in promoting integration into the community (e.g. Walsh *et al.*, 1988). People with learning disabilities are reported to have far fewer friends than their non-disabled peers (McConkey and McGinley, 1990). If people have the chance to develop and practise skills such as going to a restaurant or pub or cinema, taking part in a sport or travelling to meet a friend, with someone to help them, they may be in a position to continue the activity if the partner is not available. Exercise and sport can have positive consequences for self-image as well as health gains. The opportunity to try a range of sports and recreational activities is important (Clements, 1989). People who experience severe intellectual impairment and those who have a physical disability will benefit from exercise and leisure pursuits in which the element of risk is reasonable. Cotton (1981, 1983) stresses the value of participation and choice in a variety of activities including camping, sailing and exploration of the local environment. He believes that everyone has ability and the potential to gain from outdoor pursuits. Helping people to enjoy their leisure time is an opportunity for staff to develop their skills (Mclean, 1990).

Special care

Some developments have been thrust upon day centres as a result of changes in the types of user. The traditional response has generally been to manage these in the same way as other services. Additional special care facilities are a good example of this. As hospitals have closed or contracted, the numbers of people with profound and multiple disabilities and/or challenging behaviours requiring a day service have increased (Hughston, 1990). The most conventional method of providing these individuals with a service is to provide a special facility within the day centre. This can cause further problems with segregation (Seed, 1988). The National Development Team (1977) envisaged that special care units would become an integral part of the day centre. However, some efforts to integrate special care units within the mainstream centres have been problematic (Rose *et al.*, 1993), with staff contact being reduced after integration within the main body of the centre.

Some special care services have attempted to avoid this difficulty by having a separate, small unit based in a community facility (Taylor and Rose, 1990). This ensures staff resources are targeted at the individuals with special needs and, as the group is small and community-based, it facilitates integration. However, there are still issues of segregation that are difficult to overcome.

Services for older people with a learning disability

As the age of the general population increases and standards of health and social care improve, the numbers of people with a learning disability living into old age will also increase (Hogg *et al.*, 1988). The provision of day services to this group requires more attention. The group has been described by Sweeney and Wilson (1979) as being in 'double jeopardy'. That is, they are as economically disadvantaged and more socially isolated than other older people (Seltzer, 1985), but also suffering from the same problems of younger people with learning disabilities. As such, it has been argued that a direct application of the principles of normalization may affect this group adversely (Wolfensberger, 1985). With this in mind, a number of day service models have been developed for older people with a learning disability, which may not be directly comparable to services provided to younger people with learning disabilities. For example, a number of segregated services have specifically been developed for this client group, and they have received favourable evaluations (Carr, 1986; Foote and Rose, 1993). Other examples include pre-retirement courses aimed at preparing individuals for retirement (Haines, 1986; Cheseldine, 1989).

In the USA, there have been pioneering projects aimed at integrating older individuals with developmental disabilities into generic day services for older people (Janicki, 1991; Le Pore and Janicki, 1991; Janicki and Keefe, 1992). The expertise being developed shows clearly that effective integration into mainstream services is possible, but to develop any of these services in the UK will have considerable resource implications.

Catalysts for change

Day services are starting to change in a number of ways. It is perhaps important to consider what factors are currently facilitating change. McConkey and McGinley (1992) have listed a number of service developments that they consider to be 'The bedrock on which employment training initiatives are built and from which real jobs can become a reality'. These include normalized service settings, specific service goals, special training programmes, self-advocacy and planning for individuals.

Some of these factors – if not all of them – could be considered to have been influential in the development of all current major initiatives in day services. For example, the advent of social role valorization and the expectation for normalized service settings has meant a much greater emphasis on integration and equal opportunities. Allied to this has been the development of the growing advocacy movement (e.g. Crawley, 1988).

Individuals are increasingly speaking out on their own behalf. Advocacy, which can be defined as creating change by speaking up for one's rights, needs and wishes, has exerted an increasingly powerful influence on services in the last decade. Hersov (1992) refers to the 'indivisibility' of advocacy. It is not for an elite minority; everyone has the right to express their views or for these to be represented. The White Paper *Caring for People* (Department of Health, 1989) recognizes the importance of user participation. Griffiths (1992) believes that the care in the community changes demand 'advocacy in the broadest sense of community needs'.

Our experience as supporters of a group of self-advocates demonstrates the difficulties and rewards of trying to effect change in day services. Members of the group felt unhappy that their 'wages' of £4–5 paid at the local ATC had been withdrawn. These incentive payments had been stopped as part of a package of cuts within social services locally, prompted by government capping of community charge/council tax costs. They wished to protest about the loss of their money, which seemed to have a significance in terms of self-respect in excess of its monetary value. Members of the group had taken part in an effective protest against the closure of an ATC in another part of the county. Several group members decided that they would like to meet the director of social services in order to tell him how they felt and to ask him to restore the payments.

When the self-advocates eventually met the director after several disappointing cancellations, he explained the background to the loss of payment. Ultimately, he said that resources for the county were limited by government constraints and that a high proportion of the social services budget was allocated to the needs of people with a learning disability. When asked to restore the wages he said that it was not feasible, asking the self-advocates whether they would rather have the money or have more group homes (which are needed) provided in the area. The self-advocates had already identified the need for group homes, and indeed several were hoping to move to a supported home of their own. After discussion at the next advocacy group meeting, they decided to speak to the local MP (also a junior minister) about the issue. On voicing their views to the MP, they were told that it was a county council issue and advised to talk to the director of social services about it!

Although the objective of restoring payments was not achieved, there were nevertheless significant gains for the self-advocates in the process of attempting to change the situation. The discussions we have described did give them a greater understanding of the context of the loss of their wages. They were able to reflect on their meetings with their MP and the director of social services, both of whom did listen carefully to their views and did respond sensitively, and this is the source of some satisfaction as well as knowledge of how to take action in the future. They also raised the awareness of their MP of the aims and activities of the advocacy group.

Citizen advocacy will grow in importance in protecting the rights and needs of people with severe learning disabilites (Sutcliffe, 1990). The role of an independent representative for clients could be crucial, especially when there is a question of what is in the person's best interests. There are difficulties in the recruitment of truly independent citizen advocates.

It is clear that people who are recipients of care in the community have a wide range of needs and aspirations that cannot be met in a uniform day service. The development of human resources, and training and assessment measures available to day services, have also been influential in enabling better practice. One recent example of this is the use of a model of human occupation (e.g. Kielhofner and Nicol, 1989) by occupational therapists, which enables the therapists to assess an individual over a wide range of factors and develop appropriate individual interventions.

There are many links between these catalysts for change. Advocacy and social role valorization have been framed as a 'working alliance' between professionals and service users (Brechin and Swain, 1988). The same authors have operationalized these concepts as shared action planning (Brechin and Swain, 1987).

A note of caution

However, despite many examples of good practice and the existence of a large number of factors encouraging day service development, there are still many problems. A recent report by Mencap (1991) estimated that there is a deficit of 20 000 places in day services, and this is growing at a rate of 1000 per year. The report revealed that up to three-quarters of users had no personal programme and that people with severe learning disabilities had often received better services in hospital. Many centres were overcrowded with clients, had poor training opportunities for staff and an inability to live up to the services offered. Clearly, there is still some scope for improvement.

The advent of care management

Models of care management

We will examine the principles of care (or case) management and discuss their implications for future day services. Implementation of the National Health Service and Community Care Act 1990 is likely to exercise, via care management, a major influence on the organization and range of day provisions. Local authorities are envisaged as enablers (Audit Commission, 1986; Griffiths, 1988; Department of Health, 1989) rather than providers. Care management will be the core principle in service delivery (Malin, 1992). It is essentially a user-centred approach to service planning and delivery, in which the care manager acts as a point of contact to the user, coordinating services on the user's behalf. There is evidence that members of community teams serving people with a learning disability have used a 'case co-ordinator' model of care management with successful outcomes for clients (Ovretveit, 1991).

Individual packages of care, including day services, are designed to meet the needs and wishes of clients. The purchaser–provider divide aims to ensure that the needs of the users have priority over those of the providers. Care managers will be in a position to 'tailor' these individual programmes of care with the proviso that they have access to a range of services and the power to purchase them (Miller, 1991).

There are five distinct stages in the care management process (e.g. Wintersgill, 1991), although formulations may vary:

- *Selection*: identifying clients;
- *Assessment*: finding out what service users need and want;
- *Planning*: devising a plan in consultation with the client;
- *Implementation*: putting the agreed plan into action;
- *Monitoring/review*: checking that the services provided are as agreed and that the plan continues to be relevant to client needs. The plan will need to be reformulated if necessary.

Davies and Challis (1986) identified the following core tasks of case management: case finding and referral; assessment and selection; care planning and service packaging; monitoring and reassessment; and case closure. Use of this process in the Kent Community Care Project was designed to develop a more effective and efficient support network for elderly people at risk of premature admission to hospital for long-term care (Challis and Davies, 1986). This objective was provided by the utilization of intensive, skilled and resourceful management of cases in the context of a structure which encouraged cost-effectiveness.

The mechanisms used included the principle of small caseloads with case management targeted towards those most likely to benefit. (Only some clients need a care manager; this need may be indicated by the lack of coordination of the delivery of services by different professionals and agencies.) The whole range of social service department provision, including day care, was costed on an individual client basis. Funding was provided on the basis of a proportion, two-thirds, of the cost of residential care.

Several models of care management – a term which encompasses diverse ways of managing care – have emerged. Hunter (1988), whose primary concern was with clients with physical disabilities, discerned five:

1. The client advocacy model emphasizes the participation of clients and the accountability of the care manager to the client.

2. The care manager identifies client need when the client is unable to take part in the process, such as when a client has a profound learning disability.
3. Client advocacy within a delegated budget, as in the Kent scheme.
4. Client involvement, whereby the care manager is concerned with an individual client but the possibility exists of acting in the interests of the care group as a whole.
5. The key worker as a care manager.

Malin (1992) focuses on two broad models: 'service brokerage' and 'social entrepreneurship'. The former involves service coordination and client advocacy to some extent, whereas the latter seeks to achieve improved outcomes for clients via the use of individual budget allocations. The potential of service brokerage for people with a learning disability has been explored by means of examining its application in various forms in Canada. Brandon and Towe (1989) concluded that while service brokerage was not a panacea, it could make a substantial contribution to the empowerment of consumers.

User involvement has been a central theme of care in the community projects. A care management project for people with a learning disability in Calderdale was based on the following key tenets of the service philosophy: dignity, equality, consultation and integration (Cambridge, 1990). This had the positive effects of providing a clear value base, reducing ambiguities in practice and emphasizing service priorities and direction. It also allowed for realistic assessment of client outcomes and service achievements. Consumer perspectives were addressed formally and service users' rights protected. The disadvantages were that ideals may be difficult to attain, which may lead to disillusionment; service principles can be neutralized by competing resource demands and pressures on staff; and systems must be in place to monitor and review the effectiveness of services.

Shared action planning

This approach, proposed by Brechin and Swain (1987), which is itself a derivative of the concepts of normalization (Wolfensberger, 1972) or social role valorization (Wolfensberger, 1983) and advocacy (e.g. Williams and Schoultz, 1982), fits well with care management. It emphasizes the empowerment of the service user, whose access to services is assisted by a coordinator who is effectively carrying out care management. The coordinator relates to the client and to the client's key worker and various link workers. The key worker is in regular contact with the client and knows him or her well; link workers carry out particular interventions as part of the plan. The service user owns and directs the plan as far as possible, deciding who should be at the meeting and who gives the help needed.

Shared action planning represents a development of the individual programme plan approach (Chamberlain, 1985). In the case of severe and profound learning disabilities, the role of an independent representative (i.e. a citizen advocate) could be very significant.

Influence of care management on day services

It seems clear that social policies are geared towards future services, which are governed by the needs of individuals as identified through the assessment process. Hitherto, clients and families have generally been expected to fit into existing provisions, usually a local Adult Training Centre, which were often inappropriate or inadequate in relation to need.

Truly *individual* programmes of care for people would represent a substantial advance. Day care needs would be identified as part of a skilled overall assessment and monitored by means of regular review (Department of Health, 1992). The government vision of a mixed economy of care stresses the role of the voluntary sector in two crucial ways – as campaigner and provider. The commitment here is evinced by the fact that 34 per cent of ringfenced community care money (day care and domiciliary) allocated to local authorities must be spent within the independent sector (Yeo, 1992). The contribution to service provision of the private and voluntary sectors has been perceived as weak (Miller, 1991). The advent of the community care legislation has had an effect on day services already; the type and range of services offered has been influenced by the anticipation of its translation into action. Providers have had to consider what consumers and purchasers want from contracts. It has been suggested that larger provider organizations will be favoured because they can offer a choice to users within their services (Common and Flynn, 1992).

Those involved in setting objectives in partnership with clients and families, and in negotiating and monitoring contracts, will take account of creative initiatives like those outlined earlier in the chapter. Competent care managers will wish to ensure that service users have the opportunity, if they want it, to experience open employment and to benefit from the social networks, the self-respect and relationships which can flow from work. Therefore, we hope that 'into work' projects will grow and attract greater financial support from commissioners of services. However, these can be relatively expensive for people with greater needs, such as the need for a job coach.

The high-quality, successful day services of the future will meet the needs of *all* clients, including those from ethnic and cultural minorities. A survey in 1989 by the Social Services Inspectorate showed that few black and ethnic minority people attend day centres, even in areas where there are sizeable minority communities (Baxter et al., 1990). A good-quality day service would meet the needs of clients from minorities. This would be assisted by the employment of ethnic minority staff, so that the population of the area is reflected in the composition of the staff.

Another example of how care management could influence day services is in the area of sexuality. It is vital that people with a learning disability are aware of, and understand, their sexuality. Sensitive guidance by staff leading to greater maturity and knowledge will help to enable people to guard themselves against the risk of exploitation (Department of Health, 1992). People have been vulnerable and the risks of sexual abuse, unplanned pregnancy and HIV infection must be countered. It is acknowledged widely that agencies and organizations should have clear guidelines on sexuality, and that these will be of benefit to service users and staff (Craft, 1987). In the mixed economy of care which was heralded by *Caring for People* (Department of Health, 1989), it is crucial to ensure that policy statements and guidelines are written into contracts and agreements with the private and voluntary sector (Booth and Booth, 1992). Care management could act as a catalyst towards improved training in sexuality for users and staff.

With the implementation of community care, staff from organizations providing day care will be working with clients in a variety of settings. The trend should be away from large day centres towards greater use of mainstream resources; staff are likely to be encouraged to be more creative in their work with smaller groups of clients. Astute commissioners of day services will consider a range of leisure activities among their specifications for provider units.

It has been asserted that people who experience the greatest degree of disability are offered the least service (Mencap, 1991). Special needs units aim to meet the needs of clients with profound learning disabilities. We anticipate that people who need a greater level of support should experience different environments and activities in order to lead rewarding lives. There should be programmes of treatment and care which help service users to achieve their optimum potential (Department of Health, 1992). The Kent Project has influenced the development of day services through the care management process already. An example of the value of an independent representative might be as follows: Two day services are available and under consideration by the care manager. One service offers to provide five days of care but another will provide only three days of care for the same cost but of a perceptibly higher quality. Carers at the person's home may find the first option has an appeal, although the second may actually be in his best interests. Of course, the service user may be able to indicate his preference, but a citizen advocate's input would be valuable especially if the person does not speak or have a wide vocabulary of signs or uses another system of communication. Other difficulties may arise where there is not a truly free market in services or when some resources do not have to be paid for, such as health care.

Professionals should, in planning individual programmes of care with clients, start from an assumption that people are capable of controlling their own money (Age Concern, 1992). Choice for service users may be relatively straightforward at the local level, for example in identifying a home carer to provide support. However, at the organizational level, this is more problematic. Health authorities and private housing providers may have block contracts for the provision of day services. Block contracts of day care may be negotiated by the local authority with providers; however, money may be placed directly with care managers for 'spot contracts' to finance particular services or to fund service developments (Miller *et al.*, 1991). The Wakefield Case Management Project for people with learning disabilities appointed a project coordinator to hold the funds. This has two advantages according to Wintersgill (1991). First, care managers should not be remote from budgets because the problem of access can create difficulties in implementing clients' individual packages of care. Second, if care managers hold the budget, the competing demands of their own clients may lead to a rationing situation whereby assessments may be skewed towards existing resources rather than individual needs.

It is apposite to review the North American experience because the USA and Canada have travelled further along the contracting path. Some of the advantages and problems are becoming increasingly apparent and there are connotations for the UK. Thurlow (1992) has described the potential benefits of service brokerage, contrasting its potential for supporting clients in integrated settings with her experience of her daughter's segregated state care. Accountability of the broker to the client and family is seen as a strength. The USA is thought to be a minimum of ten years ahead of the UK in the privatization of human services. A system of specific service costing and competitive tendering operates there. The shortcomings of the contracting system in the USA have been reported. The negative consequences of the marketplace approach to human services include the fragmentation of services, difficulties in long-term planning because of the predilection for short (1–3 year) contracts, reduced staff morale, high staff turnover and low-quality output (Hadley and Ross, 1992).

Conclusion: Implications for the future

Clearly, effective care managers will have to be aware of the needs of their clients and knowledgeable about resources and relevant strategies for meeting these needs. If not, they must have access to input from those who do have the required knowledge and skills in order to assist and empower their clients. Some practitioners, notably social workers and community nurses, are already performing care management functions (e.g. Ovretveit, 1991).

At a local level, there is likely to be a major restructuring of professional roles. Social workers, as employees of the implementing authority, are seen as the natural care managers, though they are likely not to be so to the exclusion of other disciplines. It could indeed be argued that they are no better equipped to undertake the care manager role with some client groups than are colleagues who have specific training, experience and skills in working with those same groups. However, specialist knowledge of the user group is only part of the picture.

Skills in negotiating and monitoring contracts will be needed. This need may be addressed by means of inter-agency, multidisciplinary post-qualifying training in care management (Malin, 1992). It may be that, in the longer term, other professionals such as community nurses take on the role of care manager. Models of care management may vary according to local conditions. In some areas, separate care management teams may be developed. It is possible that care managers would work on complex cases with relatively small numbers of-clients.

A cornerstone of effective community care will be inter-agency cooperation. Community teams may function increasingly, post-April 1993, as commissioners of services rather than providers, according to one local proposition. This raises the question of an extended role for service workers in provider units including staff in day resources. We envisage a move towards working creatively with smaller groups in a range of mainly integrated settings. Naturally, a higher staff : client ratio and greater user choice will have cost implications.

It is in the interests of consumers that purchasers and providers of day services are able to cooperate rather than be in conflict. While those who commission services have been seen to have the financial power, it is evident that providers are closer to the service users and are, therefore, useful partners not adversaries. Day care – as with care in the community in a wider sense – should not be a purchaser versus provider battleground in which service users find themselves stranded in a political no-man's-land.

Care management has much to offer if:

1. Adequate resources are available to turn philosophy of user choice and control into reality. Statements of service principles in UK agencies do not have the legislative support of a Bill of Rights as in the USA (Dawson, 1992).
2. Clients have access to a range of good-quality services. Mencap (1991) believes that there should be: 'Statutory backing for coordinated, comprehensive day services for those who do not have a job'.
3. Clients are involved as fully as possible in their individual plans and reviews of programmes of care. Plans of care are clear and contain agreed, defined objectives of intervention.
4. Service users have access to representation by an independent advocate.

Government policy is committed to listening to clients, families, carers and advocates where appropriate (Yeo, 1992). Clients' needs and wishes should be translated into individually tailored services. Resources will be limited; however, if the limitations are too severe, the proposed changes would be negated. Optimum use must then be made of the opportunities available in order to meet clients' needs.

The development of real choice needs to be developed for *all* service users, not only those who are fortunate enough to live in an area where a progressive project exists. Without this move forward, little advantage is likely to be derived from a system of care management for day services.

Given appropriate funding, the care management system could help day services to become a rich and dynamic selection of resources. However, in a climate of severe spending restrictions and limited availability of choice, clients and care managers may have few options from which to choose. The Department of Health has announced that gaps in services or failure to meet clients' needs will not be monitored (*The Independent,* 28 January 1993). This news is disappointing, given that a fundamental principle of the new community care policy is that services should be provided on the basis of need. It is possible that, in many areas, care managers who have access to little or no alternative in service provision could continue to condemn service users to day centres which offer little variety or utility for the individual.

We hope that care management will stimulate the development of varied, high-quality day services but await the outcome with interest.

References

Age Concern (1992). *Other People's Money.* London: Age Concern.

Allen, D. (1990). Evaluation of a community-based day service for people with profound mental handicap and additional speech needs. *Mental Handicap Research,* 3(2): 179–95.

Audit Commission (1986). *Making a Reality of Community Care.* London: HMSO.

Audit Commission (1987). *Community Care: Developing Services for People with a Mental Handicap.* London: HMSO.

Baxter, C., Poonia, K., Ward, L. and Nadirshaw, Z. (1990). *Double Discrimination: Issues and Services for People with Learning Difficulties from Black and Ethnic Minority Communities.* London: King's Fund/CRE.

Bender, M. (1986). The inside out day centre. *Community Care,* 23 October, pp. 14–15.

Benz, M., Halpern, A. and Close, D. (1986). Access to day programs and leisure activities by nursing home residents with mental retardation. *Mental Retardation,* 24: 147–52.

Beyer, S. and Kilsby, M. (undated). *Methodology for the evaluation of quest.* Cardiff: Mental Handicap in Wales: Applied Research Unit.

Beyer, S., Kilsby, M. and Lowe, K. (1994). What do ATC's Offer in Wales? *Mental Handicap Research.* (In Press).

Booth, T. and Booth, W. (1992). Practice in sexuality. *Mental Handicap, 20*: 64–7.

Brandon, D. and Towe, N. (1989). *Free to Choose.* London: Community Living Monographs.

Brechin, A. and Swain, J. (1987). *Changing Relationships: Shared Action Planning for People with Learning Difficulties.* London: Harper and Row.

Brechin, A. and Swain, J. (1988). Professional and client relationships: Creating a 'working alliance' with people with learning difficulties. *Disability, Handicap and Society, 3*: 213–26.

Brown, L., Shiraga, B., Ford, A., Van Devantner, P., Nisbet, J., Loomis, R. and Sweet, M. (1987). Teaching severely handicapped adults to perform meaningful work in non-sheltered vocational environments. In Morris, R. and Blatt, B. (eds), *Perspectives in Special Education: State of the Art,* pp. 131–89. Glenview, IL: Scott, Foresman.

Browne, C. and Singh, R. (1990). 'Leisure-links'. *Mental Handicap, 18*: 35–7.

Cambridge, P. (1990). Ways forward. *Community Care,* 25 October.

Carr, P. (1986). The Falmouth Mencap Day Centre. In Wynn-Jones, A. (ed.), *Elderly People with Mental Handicap.* Taunton: Mencap.

Cassam, E. (1991). Building without bricks. *Care Weekly,* 11 January, p. 10.

Challis, D. and Davies, B. (1986). *Case Management in Community Care.* Aldershot: Gower.

Chamberlain, P. (1985). *The STEP Staff Training Package.* Rossendale: British Association for Behavioural Psychotherapy.

Cheseldine, S. (1989). Meeting the needs of older people with mental handicaps. *Mental Handicap, 17*: 96–100.

Clements, J. (1989). A psychologist's view. In Latto, K. and Norrice, B. (eds), *Give Us the Chance: Sport and Physical Recreation with People with a Mental Handicap.* London: Disabled Living Foundation.

Common, R. and Flynn, N. (1992). *Contracting for Care.* York: Joseph Rowntree Foundation.

Cotton, M. (1981). *Out of Doors with Handicapped People.* London: Souvenir Press.

Cotton, M. (1983). *Outdoor Adventure for Handicapped People.* London: Souvenir Press.

Craft, A. (1987). *Mental Handicap and Sexuality: Issues and Perspectives.* London: Costello.

Crawley, B. (1988). *The Growing Voice: A Survey of Self Advocacy Groups in Adult Training Centres and Hospitals in Great Britain.* London: CMH.

Davies, B. and Challis, D. (1986). *Matching Resources to Needs in Community Care.* Aldershot: Gower.

Dawson, C. (1992). Will Nebraska have to dance to the old tune? *Community Living,* July, pp. 8–9.

Department of Health (1989). *Caring for People: Community Care in the Next Decade and Beyond.* Cm. 849. London: HMSO.

Department of Health (1992). *Social Care for Adults with Learning Disabilities.* London: HMSO.

Floyd, M. (1990). Overcoming barriers to employment. In Dalley, G. (ed.), *Disability and Social Policy.* London: Policy Studies Institute.

Foote, K. and Rose, J. (1993). A day centre for older people with learning difficulties: The consumers' views. *Journal of Physical and Developmental Disabilities, 5*(2): 153–66.

Gathercole, C. (1987). Employment services for people with hearing impairments.

In Horobin, G. (ed.), *Why Day Care?* Research Highlights in Social Work Vol. 14. London: Jessica Kingsley.

Griffiths, R. (1988). *Community Care: Agenda for Action.* London: HMSO.

Griffiths, R. (1992). Making it happen. *Community Care,* 23 January, pp. 20–22.

Hadley, R. and Ross, I. (1992). Future imperfect. *Social Work Today,* 22 October, pp. 16–17.

Haines, C. (1986). Preparation for retirement: Workers' Educational Association pre-retirement course. In Wynn-Jones, A. (ed.), *Elderly People with Mental Handicap.* Taunton: Mencap.

Harper, G. (1989). Making each day matter. *Community Living, 3:* 11.

Hersov, J. (1992). Advocacy – issues for the 1990s. In Thompson, T. and Mathias, P. (eds), *Standards and Mental Handicap.* London: Baillière Tindall.

Hogg, J., Moss, S. and Cooke, D. (1988). *Ageing and Mental Handicap.* London: Croom Helm.

Hughston, B. (1990). Special care/special needs in day services. In Woolrych, R. (ed.), *Developing Day Services.* Ross-on-Wye: APMH.

Hunter, D. (1988). *Bridging the Gap: Case Management and Advocacy for People with Physical Handicaps.* London: King's Fund.

Jahoda, A., Cattermole, M. and Markova, I. (1989). Day services for people with mental handicap: A purpose in life. *Mental Handicap, 17*(4): 136–9.

Janicki, M.P. (1991). *Building the Future: Planning and Community Development in Ageing and Developmental Disabilities.* New York: Community Integration Project, New York State Office of Mental Retardation and Developmental Disabilities.

Janicki, M.P. and Keefe, R.M. (1992). *Integration Experiences Casebook: Programme Ideas in Ageing and Developmental Disabilities.* New York: Community Integration Project, New York State Office of Mental Retardation and Developmental Disabilities.

Jones, C. (1992). The computer workshop: Work training in a further education setting. In McConkey, R. and McGinley, P. (eds), *Innovations in Employment Training and Work for People with Learning Difficulties.* Chorley: Lisieux Hall.

Kielhofner, G. and Nicol, M. (1989). The model of human cooperation: A developing conceptual tool for clinicians. *British Journal of Occupational Therapy, 52*(6): 210–14.

King's Fund Centre (1984). *An Ordinary Working Life.* London: King's Fund.

Kregal, J. and Wehman, P. (1989). Supported employment: Promises deferred for people with severe disabilities. *Journal of the Association for Persons with Severe Handicaps, 14:* 293–303.

Le Pore, P. and Janicki, M.P. (1991). *The Wit to Win: How to Integrate Older Persons with Developmental Disabilities into Community Ageing Programmes.* New York: Community Integration Project, New York State Office of Mental Retardation and Developmental Disabilities.

Malin, N. (1992). Community care and professional directions. In Thompson, T. and Mathias, P. (eds), *Standards and Mental Handicap.* London: Baillière Tindall.

Martin, A. and Parrott, R. (1989). Out on the town. *Community Living,* April, pp. 7–8.

McConkey, R. and McGinley, P. (1990). *Innovations in Leisure and Recreation for People with a Mental Handicap.* Chorley: Lisieux Hall.

McConkey, R. and McGinley, P. (eds) (1992). *Innovations in Employment Training and Work for People with Learning Difficulties.* Chorley: Lisieux Hall.

McConkey, R., Walsh, M. and Mulcahy, M. (1981). The recreational pursuits of mentally handicapped adults. *International Journal of Rehabilitation Research,* 4: 493–9.

McConkey, R. and Murphy, R. (1989). A national survey of centres and workshops for adult persons with mental handicap. In McConkey, R. and Conliffe, C. (eds), *The Person with Mental Handicap: Preparation for an Adult Life in the Community.* Dublin: St Michael's House.

McEvoy, J., O'Mahoney, E. and Tierney, A. (1990). Parental attitudes to friendship and use of leisure by mentally handicapped persons in the community. *International Journal of Rehabilitation Research, 13*(3): 269–71.

Mclean, E. (1990). Things to do – people to see . . . *Mental Handicap, 18*: 169–71.

McLoughlin, C.S., Gardner, J.B. and Callahan, M. (1987). *Getting Employed, Staying Employed: Job Development and Training for Persons with Severe Handicaps.* Baltimore, MD: Paul Brooks.

Mencap (1991). *Empty Days . . . Empty Lives: A Report on Day Services.* London: Mencap.

Miller, C. (1991). Split vision. *Social Work Today,* 19 September, pp. 24–5.

Miller, C., Crosbie, D. and Vickery, A. (1991). *Everyday Community Care: A Manual for Managers.* London: National Institute for Social Work.

Mittler, P. (1990). Whatever happened to Pamphlet 5? In Woolrych, R. (ed.), *Developing Day Services.* Ross-on-Wye: APMH.

National Development Group for the Mentally Handicapped (1977). *Day Services for Mentally Handicapped Adults.* National Development Group Pamphlet No. 5. HMSO: London.

Nelson, I. (1990). Service without the centre. *Care Weekly,* 25 May, p. 16.

O'Brien, J. (1985). A guide to personal futures planning. In Bellamy, G. and Wilcox, B. (eds), *The Activities Catalogue: A Community Programming Guide for Youth and Adults with Severe Learning Disabilities.* Atlanta, GA: RAS.

Ovretveit, J. (1991). Case management: Notes for the perplexed. *Clinical Psychology Forum,* October, pp. 3–7.

Owens, G. and Birchenall, P. (1979). *Mental Handicap: The Social Dimensions.* Tunbridge Wells: Pitman.

Porterfield, J. and Gathercole, C. (1985). *The Employment of People with Mental Handicap: Progress Towards an Ordinary Working Life.* Project Paper No. 55. London: King's Fund.

Roberts, H. (1990). If only they could understand: Day centre workers and the parents of adults with learning difficulties. In *Social Care: Perspectives and Practice.* Coventry: Department of Applied Social Sciences, University of Warwick.

Rose, J. and Adamson, N. (1990). Investigating the problem of noise in a day centre: Are buildings designed as industrial units suitable for education and training? *British Journal of Mental Subnormality, 36*(2): 118–24.

Rose, J., Davis, C. and Gotch, L. (1993). A comparison of the care provided to profound and multiply disabled people in two different day centres. *British Journal of Developmental Disabilities, 39*(2): 83–94.

Rusch, F. (ed.) (1990). *Supported Employment: Models, Methods and Issues.* Sycamore, Illinois, Sycamore Publishing.

Seed, P. (1988). *Day Care at the Crossroads.* Tunbridge Wells: Costello.

Seltzer, M.M. (1985). Informal support of ageing mentally retarded persons. *American Journal of Mental Retardation, 90*: 259–65.

Shafer, M.S., Wehman, P., Kregal, J. and West, M. (1990). National supported employment initiative: A preliminary analysis. *American Journal of Mental Retardation, 95*: 316–27.

Shanly, A. and Rose, J. (1993). A consumer survey of adults with learning difficulties currently doing work experience: Their satisfaction with work and wishes for the future. *Mental Handicap Research, 6*(3): 153–262.

Shearer, A. (1986). *Building a Community for People with Mental Handicaps*. London: CMH.

Sikking, M. (1986). *Co-ops with a Difference: Co-ops Employing People with Special Needs*. London: ICOM Publications.

Social Services Inspectorate (1989). *Inspection of Day Services*. London: Department of Health.

Sutcliffe, J. (1990). *Adults with Learning Difficulties: Education for Choice and Empowerment*. London: NIACE.

Sweeney, D.P. and Wilson, T.Y. (eds) (1979). *The Plight of Ageing and Aged Developmentally Disabled Persons in Mid America*. Logan, UT: Exceptional Child Center, Utah State University.

Taylor, T. and Rose, S. (1990). Creating quality day services. *Nursing, 4*(18): 32–6.

Thurlow, J. (1992). My journey through despair led to the Holy Grail. *Community Living*, July, pp. 12–14.

Walsh, P., Coyle, K. and Lynch, C. (1988). The Partners Project. *Mental Handicap, 16*: 122–5.

Wertheimer, A. (1985). *Going to Work: Employment Opportunities for People with Mental Handicaps in Washington State, USA*. London: HMSO. Campaign for People with a Mental Handicap.

Wertheimer, A. (1987). Towards a normal working life. *Community Living*, April, pp. 8–9.

Wertheimer, A. (1992). Give us the tools. *Community Care*, 6 February, pp. 16–17.

Whelan, E. and Speake, B. (1977). *Adult Training Centres in England and Wales: Report of the First National Survey*. Manchester: Revelland George.

Williams, P. and Schoultz, B. (1982). *We Can Speak for Ourselves*. London: Souvenir Press.

Wintersgill, C. (1991). Separate identities. *Social Work Today*, 17 October, p. 22.

Wolfensberger, W. (1972). *The Principle of Normalization in Human Services*. Toronto: NIMR.

Wolfensberger, W. (1983). Social role valorization: A proposed new term for the principle of normalization. *Mental Retardation*, December, pp. 234–9.

Wolfensberger, W. (1985). An overview of social role valorization and some reflections on elderly mentally retarded persons. In Janicki, M.P. and Wisniewski, H.M. (eds), *Ageing and Developmental Disabilities: Issues and Trends*. Baltimore, MD: Paul Brooks.

Woolf, J. (1990). How can we help people to get employed and stay employed? In Woolrych, R. (ed.), *Developing Day Services*. Ross-on-Wye: APMH.

Woolrych, R. (ed.) (1990). *Developing Day Services*. Ross-on-Wye: APMH.

Yeo, T. (1992). Converting rights into realities from the perspective of health and social services. Speech to the Mencap Conference on *Positive Images: Positive Action*. London, October.

11 Domiciliary services

Aileen McIntosh and Andy Alaszewski

Introduction

Caring for People (Department of Health, 1989: para. 1.11) places as a priority
'promoting the development of domiciliary, day and respite services to
enable people to live in their own homes wherever possible and sensible',
stating that existing funding structures have worked against the development of such services: 'In future, the Government will encourage the
targeting of home-based services on those people whose need for them
is greatest'. The future development depends both on the availability of
staff and the success achieved by social services departments (SSDs) in
contracting-out domiciliary services. A report published by the Audit Commission (1992) drew attention to the difficulties that can arise if health
and social care are not clearly defined, arguing that district health authorities need to provide extra nursing support for people leaving residential
care: currently this is seen as a local authority issue. The roles of home
help and district nurse in community care continue to change. Tim Booth's
coverage of a survey conducted in partnership with the National Council
of Domiciliary Care Services (Joint Unit for Social Services Research and
Booth, 1990) showed that there is a long way to go before anything approaching a contract culture takes root in the domiciliary field. Only 23
(21 per cent) of the 109 authorities who responded reported having contracts with independent suppliers for the provision of domiciliary services.
The absence of effective proposals to enhance domiciliary care has
highlighted the wide diversity of costs, whereas neglect of the 'economies
of scale' argument in translating costs from residential services has resulted
in failure to establish realistic alternative costs.

In this chapter, we examine the development of official policy in relationship to families caring for children who have a learning disability and use
findings from our research into families in North Humberside to explore
the extent to which changes in official policy have begun to percolate

through to these families, illustrating their need for more domiciliary and other forms of provision. In our discussion of official policy, we will show that attitudes to, and the expected role of, families have changed radically this century. At the beginning of the century, families were seen as the problem and institutional care was developed as the solution. In the 1950s, there was a role reversal, institutions had become the problem and families the solution – the centrepiece of the new policy of community care.

Despite changes in attitudes and the changing rhetoric of official policy, our studies in North Humberside demonstrate that little has altered in the reality of day-to-day care. In the last decade, families – and particularly mothers – have provided the bulk of community care. Although some areas of support have improved, the underlying picture remains much the same – support from services remains minimal.

The development of official policy: Policing the family

People with a learning disability only became the subject of official policy, and 'visible' to policy makers as a distinctive group with needs that the state could and should cater for, at the beginning of the twentieth century (Alaszewski and Ong, 1991). The 1913 Mental Deficiency Act established a legislative and administrative framework for the care of 'mental defectives'. This framework was developed during a period of social and political turbulence in which competition and conflict between the imperial states of Europe focused official attention on the quality of the population. 'Mental defectives' were seen as a major handicap in that competition, as they were seen as undermining the quality of the population.

> Many persons now classified as imbeciles and the majority of those now classified as feeble minded are able to live in the general community with relatives or friends and are accustomed to mix and work with other people; if their relatives or friends die or become unable to give them a home any longer, they need to be provided with a home by some public authority.
>
> (Royal Commission, 1957: para. 592)

The Commission recast the relationship between agencies and families. Although there remained a vestigial supervisory role, the main emphasis was on supporting families: 'When a patient is living with his own family, one of the most important functions of the social worker or mental welfare officers is to advise his family and to try to ensure that they understand his needs and difficulties' (Royal Commission, 1957: para. 669).

Policy statements in the 1960s and 1970s increasingly emphasized the central role of families in providing care. For example, the Ministry of Health's (1963) overview of the development of local authority health and welfare services endorsed the role of the family in the following way:

It is usually best for the mentally disordered person in the community, whether adult or child, to live at home where this is possible . . . the services provided inside and outside the home can
improve an unfavourable situation and make it unnecessary to seek
an alternative.

(Ministry of Health, 1963: 25)

The 1971 White Paper, *Better Services for the Mentally Handicapped*, saw the
family as the best place for providing care: 'Each handicapped person
should live with his own family as long as this does not impose an undue
burden on them or him, and he and his family should receive full advice
and support' (DHSS, 1971: 9). The White Paper set the tone for the subsequent policy debate. Family care was not only seen as the best form of
care, it was also the main locus of care. However, the report recognized
that most families did not receive adequate support:

Most parents are devoted to their handicapped children and wish to
care for them and to help them to develop their full potential. About
80 per cent of severely handicapped children and 40 per cent of
severely handicapped adults – and a higher proportion of the more
mildly handicapped – live at home. Their families need advice and
many forms of help, most of which at present are rarely available.

(DHSS, 1971: para. 20)

Families have been centre-stage in virtually all the major policy statements since the White Paper. For example, a 1980 Department of Health
review of service for people with learning disabilities stated: 'The emphasis
of both health and social services is increasingly on maintaining the child
within his own family wherever possible, by providing practical help,
counselling and periods of short-term residential care' (para. 2.35). This
view was reiterated in the government's response to the 1985 Social Services
Select Committee Report on Community Care: 'It has recently been restated
that government policy is to "enable each mentally handicapped person
to live with his [or her] own family, if this does not impose an undue
burden"' (DHSS, 1985). In *Caring for People* (Department of Health, 1989),
the blueprint for the development of community care, the government
has a clear perception of the importance of informal care: 'The Government
acknowledges that the great bulk of community care is provided by friends,
family and neighbours' (p. 4).

The parallel and complementary theme in most of these policy statements
is that, although families need considerable support in providing care,
they rarely receive it. The 1981 government handbook of policies and
priorities, *Care in Action*, described the pressure on families in the following
way: 'The scale of support that some people require if they are to live at
home is considerable, and the burden on their families can be heavy'

(DHSS, 1981: para. 4.10). However, the Department of Health review of services for people with a learning disability accepted that families were not receiving adequate support: 'When studies of community care are reported they have been disquieting and suggest that many families are not receiving the help they need' (DHSS, 1980: para. 2.9).

The Social Services Select Committee, in its 1985 review of community care, drew attention to the major flaw in government policy. Although families played a central role in providing community care, the problems associated with closing institutions tended to preoccupy policy makers, and therefore families have tended not to attract attention nor resources:

> Many witnesses have told the Committee of the sometimes intolerable burden of care that is placed on the families of mentally ill and mentally handicapped people who are living at home. Constant demands may exact a heavy toll on families, and particularly on parents. According to the Social Policy Unit at the University of York – "The community care of young mentally and multiply impaired young adults involves arduous and unremitting physical work and watchfulness, similar to the care and supervision needed by a young child but extending over a lifetime and becoming increasingly onerous as both parents and the young person grow older . . . the burden of care falls largely on the young person's mother and results in marked financial, physical and emotional costs" . . . Community care depends heavily at the end of the day on relatives caring for their own family members. There is a danger that the establishment of new and expensively staffed services will produce a continuation of the present relative neglect of families caring in the community, to their personal and financial cost.
> (House of Commons Social Services Select Committee, 1985)

There has been growing recognition in the last twenty years that families will only be able to act as the cornerstone of community care if they receive adequate support. In the 1980s, this concern began to affect the services provided by local agencies. In the next section, we explore the impact of these changes on one group of families in the North of England.

Supporting families

In this section, we discuss the findings of a study which was conducted between 1989 and 1990 of 51 families in North Humberside. The study was designed to monitor the impact which changes in service provision were having on families caring for children with a learning disability. The impetus for the study came from a workshop for local service providers which was held at the University of Hull in 1987. At this workshop, we reported on the findings of our earlier Humberside study. We had found that mothers caring for children with a learning disability and their families received minimal support from formal services:

> Welfare provisions tended to be oriented towards dealing with short term crises and emergencies rather than coping with the long term needs of mothers who care for their severely handicapped children. For these mothers community care can seem an abstract and meaningless concept. They do not want the traditional segregated services of the large scale institution nor do they want piecemeal, haphazard contact with a constantly changing group of generic workers. Like the professionals they want to prevent the development of a crisis and therefore they want co-ordinated specialist services that operate within the framework of generic services and which provide them with sensitive and appropriate practical help.
>
> (Ayer and Alaszewski, 1986: 195–6)

Several of the senior local service providers were adamant that major changes had taken place in the organization and delivery of services, especially health and social services, since we had undertaken our first study and its findings were no longer relevant. These changes included the development of improved ways of disclosing the nature of a child's disability to his or her parents, improvements in providing advice to parents and the development of community mental handicap teams. In their view, these changes amounted to a comprehensive package of support which was transforming the experience of family care and the relationship between the families and professionals.

We therefore decided to conduct a second follow-up survey of families in North Humberside to examine the impact of the changes in the 1980s on family support. We revisited 26 of the families in the original study to see how they were experiencing the changes and visited 25 new families that had started their career as carers in the 1980s. We will organize our discussion of the findings of our survey into two sections: the first will deal with the role of specific services, and the second will deal with parents' perceptions of professionals.

Services for families

Initial contact: Identifying a special need   For most parents, their contact with specialist services came when the nature and extent of their child's disability was first disclosed. Although good models have been developed for discussing the nature and extent of a child's disability with parents (see, e.g. Cunningham *et al.*, 1984), most studies indicate continuing problems with this crucial phase in the parents' relationship with their child and with the services (see, e.g. Glendinning, 1983; Murdoch, 1984; Jupp, 1987; Quine and Pahl, 1987; Nursey *et al.*, 1991). Plank's (1987) study showed that there appears to be little consistency in practice of the way disclosure is handled by health authorities.

We also found that these initial encounters with services and profession-als at the time of disclosure were frequently unsatisfactory. Even where parents had been in contact with the same agency, the way they were handled and told depended on the procedures used by the doctor or other professional who talked to them. Many parents clearly remained very upset and disturbed by the ways in which they were told, even parents who had had the opportunity to discuss the issue in the new child clinics. One mother described her experience: 'He just held Christopher up by his feet and said, you know it was just as if he was a piece of meat, "don't expect anything from him because he'll never be like your daughter".' In some cases, the parents felt they had been left to work it out for themselves from various hints and clues given by professionals. As one mother said: '. . . they said that she had problems with her speech, and other things but they didn't define it . . . they didn't say what disability it was or anything and I still don't know'.

The ways in which parents were treated during the disclosure process appeared to have an important impact on their subsequent attitude to services. It tended to set the tone for subsequent parent–professional re-lationships. After their encounter with services and professionals at the time of disclosure, many parents assumed, often quite rightly, that they would have a struggle to obtain information, to get professionals to take them seriously and to achieve any type of partnership in the care of their child.

Finding out about services   Parents cannot use services if they do not know that they exist or do not know how to access them. As the National De-velopment Team (1982: 30) noted: 'Unless families are told of the exist-ence of services they are unlikely to become aware of them'. A repetitive theme in the literature is that parents often do not know about services, and therefore cannot make use of them. Our study indicated that among parents in North Humberside, there has been a slight improvement in knowledge about allowances and services for parents in this area, when compared with Ayer and Alaszewski's study in the late 1970s. The vast majority of information about services and allowances had come from other parents, television, newspapers and the like. This was true for par-ents both in regular contact with professionals and those who were not.

However, there was at the same time too much information about some aspects of services. For example, new benefit books were often accom-panied by a shower of leaflets and booklets on national benefits. This information was often irrelevant or duplicated information. Parents wanted and found it difficult to obtain relevant information about local services such as contact names. Although one of the local Community Mental

Handicap Teams (CMHT) had produced a guide to local services, none of the parents we interviewed had a copy. It seemed to be restricted to local service providers.

It was frustrating for some parents to know that in theory certain services were available, for example home sitting, but for all intents and purposes they were unavailable as such services seemed to be allocated by local service providers to other clients.

Receiving services: The Community Mental Handicap Teams Multidisciplinary teams such as CMHTs represent a major innovation and service development of the 1980s. The majority of the families (*n* = 43; 84 per cent) in the North Humberside study were aware of the teams, although only thirty (59 per cent) knew them by that name. The majority of respondents knew of community nurses and were aware that community nurses were part of a team. Most parents were in contact with an integrated team (McGrath, 1991), which included social workers, community nurses, other health professionals and service organizers. However, their contact was usually with only one team member, often a community nurse, and they did not use this point of contact as a way of accessing the resources of the whole team. The teams did not achieve the National Development Team (1982: 11) objective of providing a coordinated service.

One of the reasons for the failure of the CMHTs to fulfil this role may be simply that they were victims of their own success. The CMHTs were widely promoted and parents seemed to have developed high expectations of their services. They tended to be disappointed by the reality of the finite resources available to the teams.

Receiving services: Respite care Parents of children with a learning disability are unable to look forward to a reduction in the level of care. Indeed, as their children grow older, the level of care may increase. Respite care can be one way for parents and other family members to have a break from the demanding routines involved in caring for a disabled relative. It also allows parents time to spend with other children, who may not get as much attention when the disabled sibling is at home. It is usually considered as having a positive effect on the family. However, recent findings (Gerard, 1990; Jawed *et al.*, 1992) have pointed out that in some instances, albeit a minority, there can be negative effects. Gerard (1990: 155) has argued that 'a sizeable minority of carers and their children seem to encounter problems with respite care, and they may conclude that, for some people, respite services have a negligible or even detrimental, effect on quality of life'.

We found instances when parents were apprehensive or had reservations about respite care. Some reservations were based on previous experiences of respite care, sometimes many years ago in old mental handicap hospitals.

Others reasons for apprehension were due to parents worrying about the child during the period of respite. Some parents did not want to use respite care because they did not feel it provided a satisfactory standard of care in a suitable location and that their child did not benefit from it. One mother described the reasons why she did not use a particular facility in the following way: 'Kenneth has to gain a lot by these days and I don't think he did that day. The people that he was with were far too severely handicapped for him to gain anything, so he never went back.' The dilemma facing many mothers when deciding whether to use respite care was clearly identified by Hubert (1991: 112) in her study of twenty families: 'It is difficult for mothers, especially, to balance their own needs for sleep, for time alone or with their husbands, against their child's need for love and comfort, familiar faces and clean nappies'.

The majority of parents in our study had and did use respite care and found it invaluable. For school age children, most respite care was spent at hostels attached to the special schools that the children attended. This was valued by parents because it provided a certain degree of continuity and parents had confidence in the care provided in the school.

Receiving services: Education   All the children and young adults being looked after in our study were attending special schools, or had done so in the past. The parents tended to think that their children had done better at special schools than they would have done in mainstream schools. Many parents were also concerned about the educational aspects of their child's schooling. Parents no longer simply saw schooling primarily in terms of being a child-minding service during the week. Most wanted, expected and felt that their child had benefited from school, in areas such as reading, writing and numeracy, as well as social and life skills. Parents were also concerned about the friendships that their children would have, or might not have, made in a mainstream school. Almost all the parents (94 per cent) in our study thought that special schools should exist.

Parents were unhappy with the isolationist aspect of special schools, and most favoured the option of having a special unit attached to a mainstream school:

> I believe in partial integration, really I don't believe in integration, I don't think it would do either type of child any good to be totally integrated. I think it will be disruptive for the normal children, and I don't think the handicapped child will benefit. What I think is probably the best method is to have a unit in a school but no way total integration.

Overall, while parents were happy with special schools, this may have more to do with them being unconvinced and unsure that integration would work.

Separate schooling is one of the most visible ways in which people with learning disabilities are still treated separately, and often leads to the involvement of specialized professionals, and hence specialist services, with the family.

General assessment of services We asked parents what their overall opinion of services was. Forty-nine per cent felt services were good, 14 per cent felt they were poor, 18 per cent said they were neither good nor bad, and 20 per cent said they did not use any services and therefore did not offer an opinion. When parents thought they were good, or just alright, they often attached a qualification, such as: 'They're OK, the services available are OK, but there aren't enough of them, that's the biggest criticism of them really'.

We also asked parents who had taken part in the earlier study if they thought that services had improved, stayed the same or got worse. Of those twenty-six parents, sixteen (62 per cent) said they had improved, eight (31 per cent) said they had stayed the same and two (8 per cent) said they had got worse. Comments when parents were not happy with the services were more abundant. Several of the parents who had taken part in the earlier study pointed out that while the services had improved, their needs had also increased, so that the services remained inadequate. One mother said: 'They've probably improved. They've altered I think, altered greatly . . . But whether it's an improvement I really don't know'.

On the whole, parents seemed to feel that services were alright if they could find out about them, but resources were not available in sufficient quantity to fully compensate for having to care for a child with a learning disability. Service innovations such as CMHTs and more specifically community nurses were seen as very valuable and helpful. There have been some improvements in the awareness of what was available. Some services, such as respite care, have changed, and parents' views about whether this is for the better are varied. The impression that parents gave in their views of statutory services is that overall things have got better since the last study, but there is still a long way to go.

Families and professionals

The experiences of services usually depends on contacts parents have with individual service providers, as Lloyd-Bostock (1976) has argued. How parents and professionals see each other will obviously have far-reaching effects on the provision of services, and how they are provided. Twigg (1989) has suggested that professionals can relate to or treat carers in one of three ways: carers as resources, carers as co-workers, or carers as co-clients. The majority of parents in our study still fell into the carers as resources model, as far as many services are concerned. Many services were still on a crisis intervention footing, only available when that resource, the carer, was for whatever reason no longer able to cope. For some parents, and with some services, other models prevailed. In some instances, the relationship that parents had with their community nurse might be better described as following the carers as co-clients typology.

Professionals still tended to adopt the role of 'expert' (Appleton and Mincham, 1991). This expert role is based on the traditional medical model – professionals assess and treat a particular problem without necessarily making careful reference to parental wishes, views and feelings. Negotiation between the parents and professionals with respect to assessment and treatment objectives is given a relatively low priority. In turn, parents may be reluctant to question the professionals' apparent objectives. A particular problem is the narrow focus of professional interest and the lack of fit between parental goals and professional goals. As a result, the relationship between parents and professionals is often difficult.

Much of the literature and research in the field of learning disability focuses on the problems of having a child, or family member, who is seen as having needs that require specialist help. Dyson (1986: 80) has challenged this view:

> ... the problems facing parents of mentally-handicapped children are simply the ordinary problems of bringing up a child writ large. Practical difficulties are not distinct problems which suddenly appear when a family has a handicapped child. Rather, they are the "normal" problems of parents bringing up their children, only extended over a longer period of time, and more frequently complicated by there being a number of problems occurring together.

Some groups such as the Campaign for Mentally Handicapped People (now Values into Action) have argued that all services for people with a learning disability should be provided within the framework of generic services available to all citizens (Tyne and Wertheimer, 1980). Specialized services can be thought of as existing only for people with disabilities, in contrast to generic services which are available to everyone. The provision of separate services, it is suggested, in itself contributes to the idea that the recipients are somehow different. Instead, it is suggested that generic services should be used. In 1992, Wickham and Blackmore presented findings that suggested that the majority of parents in their study were in favour of generic services. There were different levels of support for the idea across different income and education levels. We asked the parents in our study whether they felt there 'should be special services for people with a mental handicap'. All the parents felt there should be such services.

Some parents gave general reasons ('Yes, because their needs are different to ordinary people. They need different sorts of things'), whereas others gave more specific reasons. One mother, for example, mentioned the provision and use of special dental services: 'If you've got to use an ordinary doctor or dentist they haven't got the know how to cope or deal with anybody like Julian. You couldn't take him to an ordinary dentist because he wouldn't know where to start'. Some parents cited problems they encountered with societal reactions and the support which specialist services could provide: '. . . people can be extremely rude and not very helpful at all . . . and then you turn to the special services'. Some parents felt that practitioners in specialist services developed specialist expertise: 'There are certain areas where you feel a lot more confident if you know that someone has that specialist knowledge'. The parents we interviewed did not see it as an 'either/or' situation. They wanted to use both generic and specialist services as appropriate.

The main problems related not to who provided a service, but how it was provided and in particular the relationship they had with the specific professional. The most common problem was a lack of an effective, and close, parent–professional relationship. However, occasionally, a parent–professional relationship that was too friendly also posed problems. Parents could experience a major loss when staff changed. A close relationship meant that parents sometimes felt unable to voice grievances about services as such complaints could be seen as a complaint against a friend.

Conclusions

There has been a major transformation in official thinking about the role of families in providing care for people with learning disabilities. Unless effective support is provided for families, then community care is little more than a cynical cost-cutting exercise in which the responsibility of care is shifted from the state to the family and very little effective support is provided for families.

Families are unlikely to receive more effective support unless there is a radical change in the role of professionals and their attitudes to families. A move towards partnership is required. This will require considerable change on the part of professionals to value and accept the knowledge of families. It also requires a greater awareness on the part of parents of what constitutes service provision. Professionals have a key role in providing parents with information about and explanations of the services which they can use. The implementation of the National Health Service and Community Care Act 1990, with its emphasis on assessment, care management and the greater responsibilities that local authorities have, should mean a move towards a greater degree of partnership between parents and professionals. However, past experience has shown that during a major restructuring of services, considerable time and resources are devoted to the process of change and very little may percolate through to families. As Hubert has pointed out when discussing the Griffiths Report on Community Care (1988), the need is for quick and targeted action:

The quick and full implementation of these recommendations by Government is the only spark of hope for the twenty young adults in this book – and for their parents, who have so clearly and consistently expressed their dissatisfaction with the current provision of services . . . the exceptional nature of the problems confronted by such parents and their children are unlikely to be met by more general strategies and intentions – they demand specific action.

(Hubert, 1991)

There also has to be a necessary shift in emphasis to help achieve a greater degree of congruence between rhetoric and reality. Simply repeating in policy document after policy document that support for families is crucial to the success of community care does not create an effective service. Recent changes in policy and legislation continue to be based on the rhetoric that the family supported by services is the basis of community care; in reality, the family provides the majority of care with minimal support.

References

Alaszewski, A. and Ong, B.N. (1991). From consensus to conflict: The impact of sociological ideas on policy for people with a mental handicap. In Baldwin, S. and Hattersley, J. (eds), *Mental Handicap: Social Science Perspectives*. London: Routledge/Tavistock.

Appleton, P.L. and Mincham, P.E. (1991). Models of parent partnership and child development centres. *Child: Care, Health and Development, 17*(1): 27–38.

Audit Commission (1992). *Homeward Bound: A New Course for Community Health.* London: HMSO.

Ayer, S. and Alaszewski, A. (1986). *Community Care and the Mentally Handicapped: Services for Mothers and Mentally Handicapped Children*, 2nd edn. London: Croom Helm.

Cunningham, C.C., Morgan, P.A. and McGucken, R.B. (1984). Down's syndrome: Is dissatisfaction with disclosure of diagnosis inevitable? *Developmental Medicine and Child Neurology, 26*: 33–9.

Department of Health (1963). *Health and Welfare: The Development of Community Care.* London: HMSO.

Department of Health (1989). *Caring for People: Community Care in the Next Decade and Beyond.* Cm. 849. London: HMSO.

Department of Health and Social Security (1971). *Better Services for the Mentally Handicapped.* Cmnd. 4683. London: HMSO.

Department of Health and Social Security (1980). *Mental Handicap: Progress, Problems and Priorities.* London: HMSO.

Department of Health and Social Security (1981). *Care in Action.* London: HMSO.

Department of Health and Social Security (1985). *Government Response to the Second Report from the Social Services Committee, 1984–85 Session: Community Care – With*

Special Reference to Adult Mentally Ill and Mentally Handicapped People. Cmnd 9674. London: HMSO.

Dyson, S. (1986). Professionals, mentally handicapped children and confidential files. *Disability, Handicap and Society, 1*(1): 73–87.

Gerard, K. (1990). Economic evaluation of respite care for children with mental handicaps: A preliminary analysis of problems. *Mental Handicap, 18*: 150–55.

Glendinning, C. (1983). *Unshared Care: Parents and Their Disabled Children.* London: Routledge and Kegan Paul.

Griffiths, R. (1988). *Community Care: Agenda for Action.* London: HMSO.

House of Commons Social Services Select Committee (1985). *Second Report, 1984–85: Community Care.* London: HMSO.

Hubert, J. (1991). *Home-bound: Crisis in the Care of Young People with Severe Learning Difficulties. A Story of Twenty Families.* London: King's Fund.

Jawed, S.H., Krishnan, V.H.R. and Oliver, B.E. (1992). Respite care for children with mental handicap: Service evaluation and profile of children. *British Journal of Mental Subnormality, 38*(1): 15–23.

Joint Unit for Social Services Research and Booth, T.A. (1990). *Better Lives: Changing Services for People with Learning Difficulties.* Sheffield: University of Sheffield.

Jupp, S. (1987). Breaking the news: A way of telling parents their newborn child is handicapped. *Mental Handicap, 15*(1): 8–11.

Lloyd-Bostock, S. (1976). Parents' experiences of official help and guidance in caring for a mentally handicapped child. *Child: Care, Health and Development, 2*: 325–38.

McGrath, M. (1991). *Whatever Happened to Teamwork? Reflections on CMHTs.* Bangor: Centre for Social Policy Research and Development, University of Wales.

Mental Deficiency Committee (1929). *Report, Part III: The Adult Defective.* London: HMSO.

Murdoch, J.C. (1984). Immediate post-natal management of the mothers of Down's syndrome and spina bifida children in Scotland, 1971–1981. *Journal of Mental Deficiency Research, 28*: 67–72.

National Development Team for the Mentally Handicapped (1982). *Third Report: 1979–1981.* London: HMSO.

Nursey, A., Rohde, J.R. and Farmer, R.D.T. (1991). Ways of telling new parents about their child and his or her mental handicap: A comparison of doctors' and parents' views. *Journal of Mental Deficiency Research, 35*(1): 48–57.

Plank, M. (1987). *Begin at the Beginning: An Enquiry into Early Support for Families with a Handicapped Baby.* London: Campaign for Mentally Handicapped People.

Quine, L. and Pahl, J. (1987). First diagnosis of severe handicap: A study of parental reactions. *Developmental Medicine and Child Neurology, 29*: 232–42.

Royal Commission on the Law Relating to Mental Illness and Mental Deficiency (1957). *Report.* Cmnd 169. London: HMSO.

Twigg, J. (1989). Models of carers: How do social care agencies conceptualise their relationship with informal carers? *Journal of Social Policy, 18*(1): 53–66.

Tyne, A. and Wertheimer, A. (1980). *Even Better Services? A Critical Review of Mental Handicap Policies in the 1970s.* London: Campaign for Mentally Handicapped People.

Index